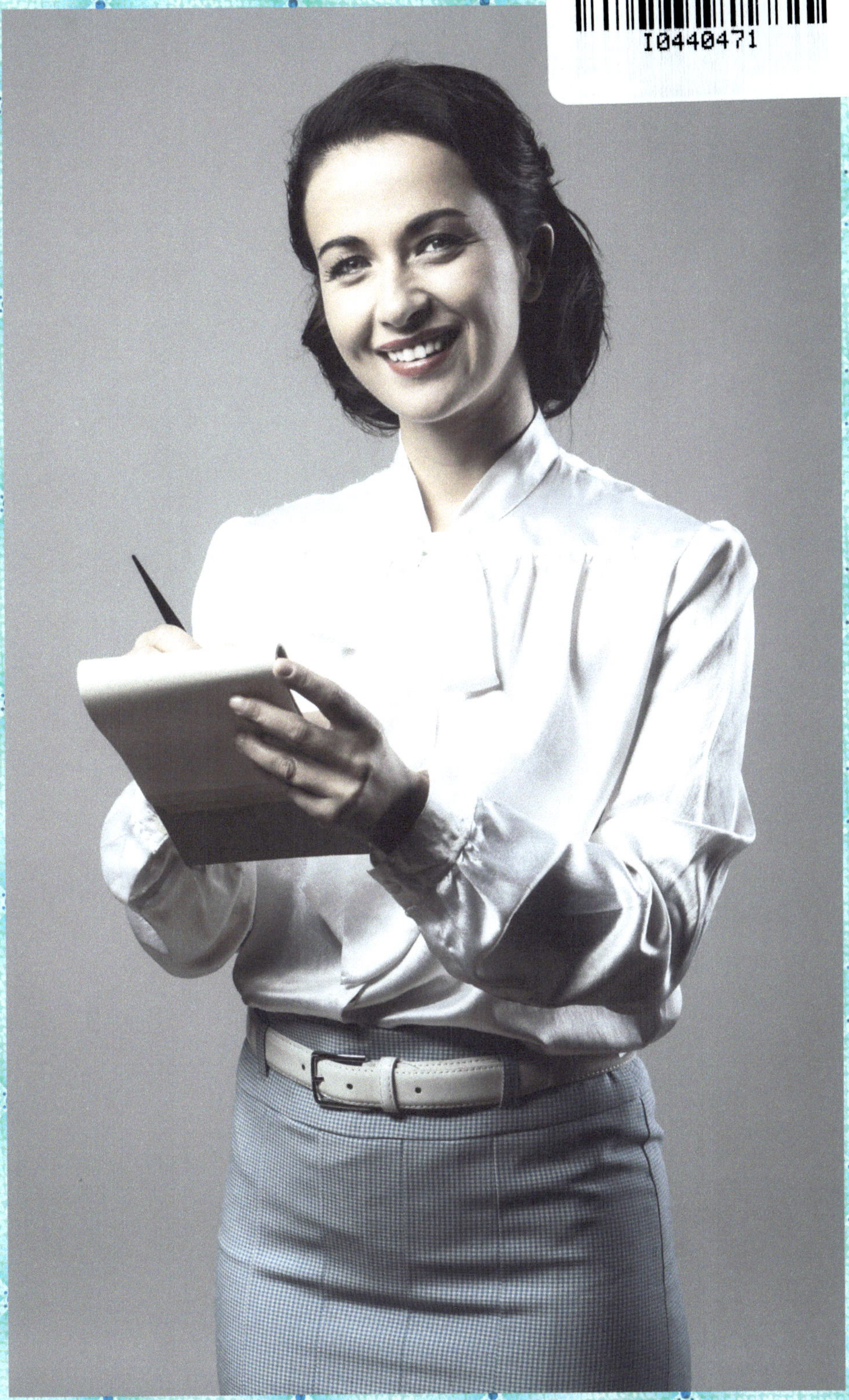

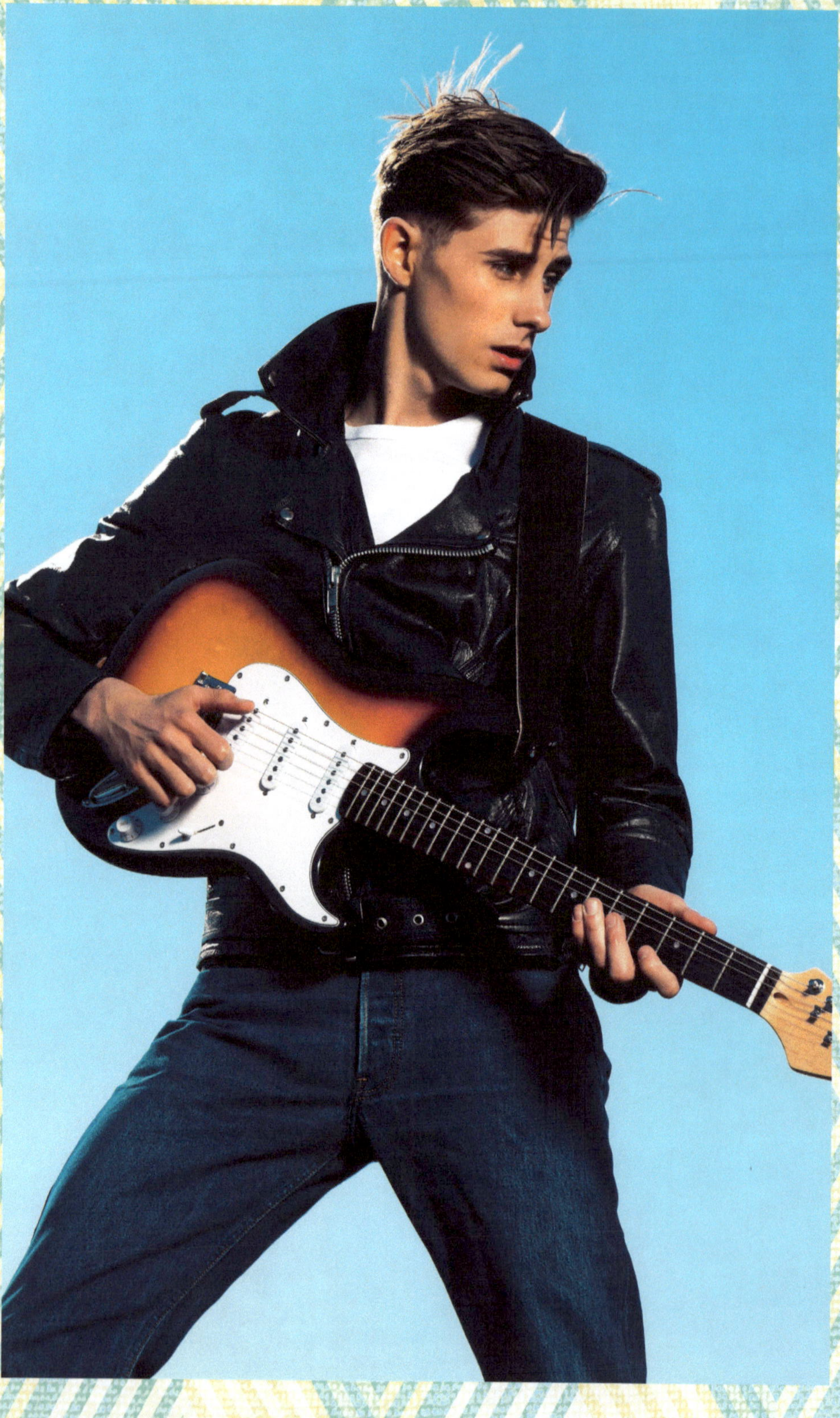

ADULT PICTURE BOOK OF
1950s Memories

FASHION AND CLOTHES

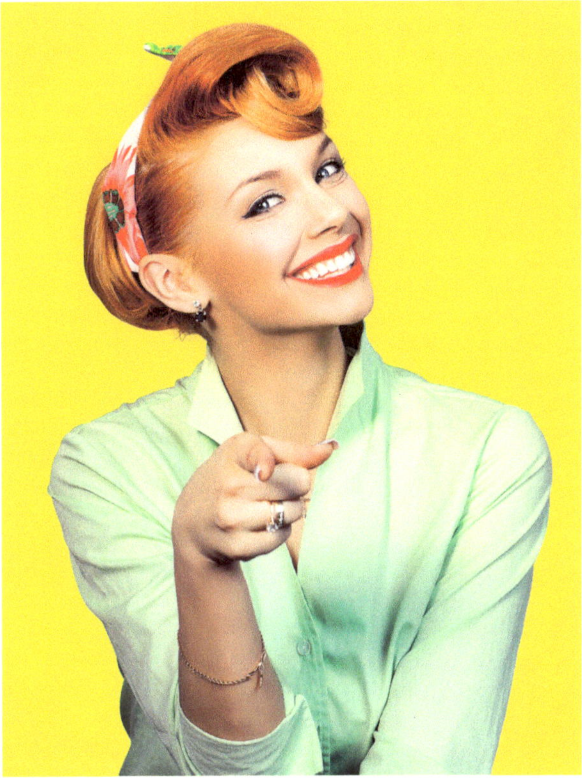

Spring Lane Press

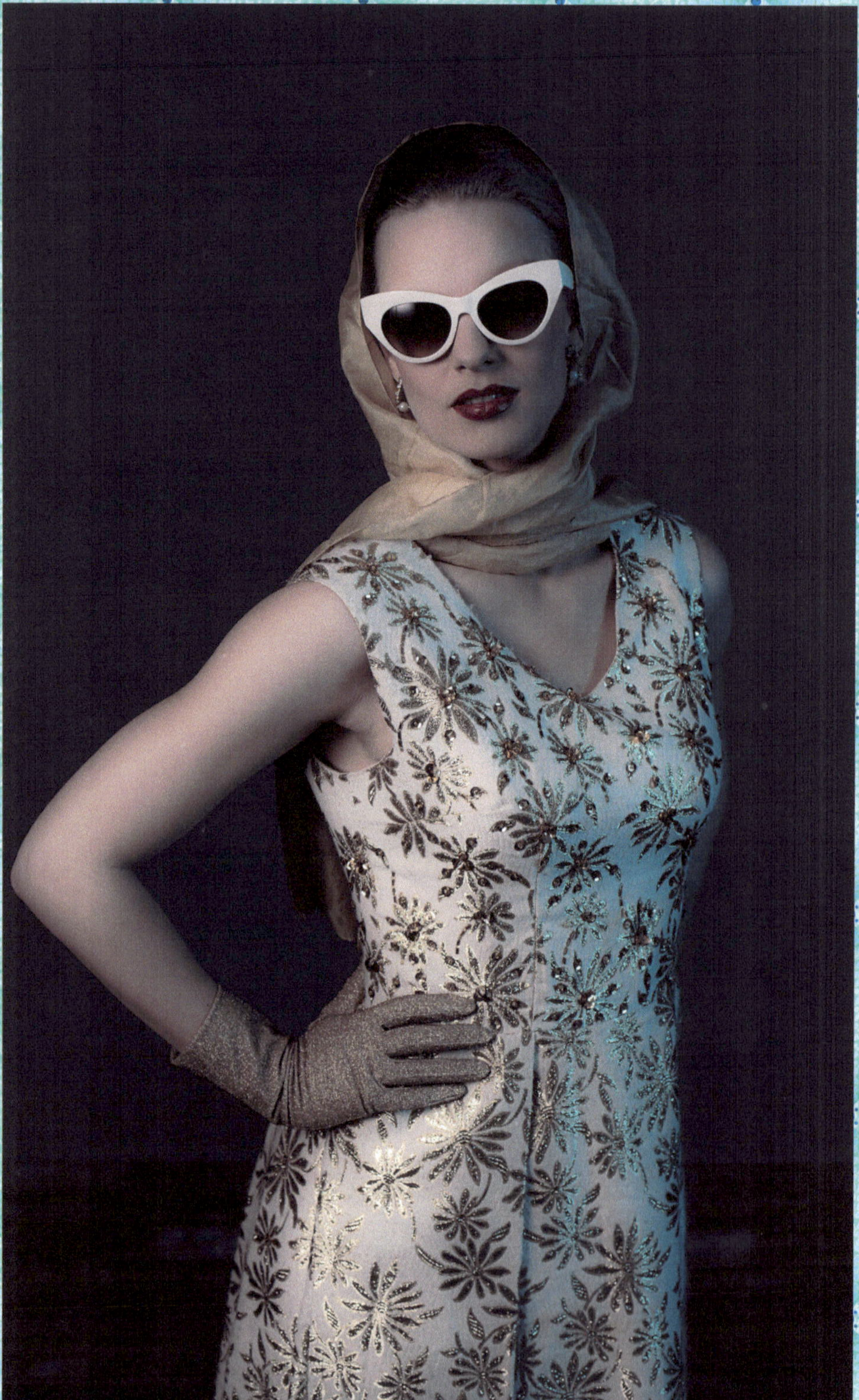

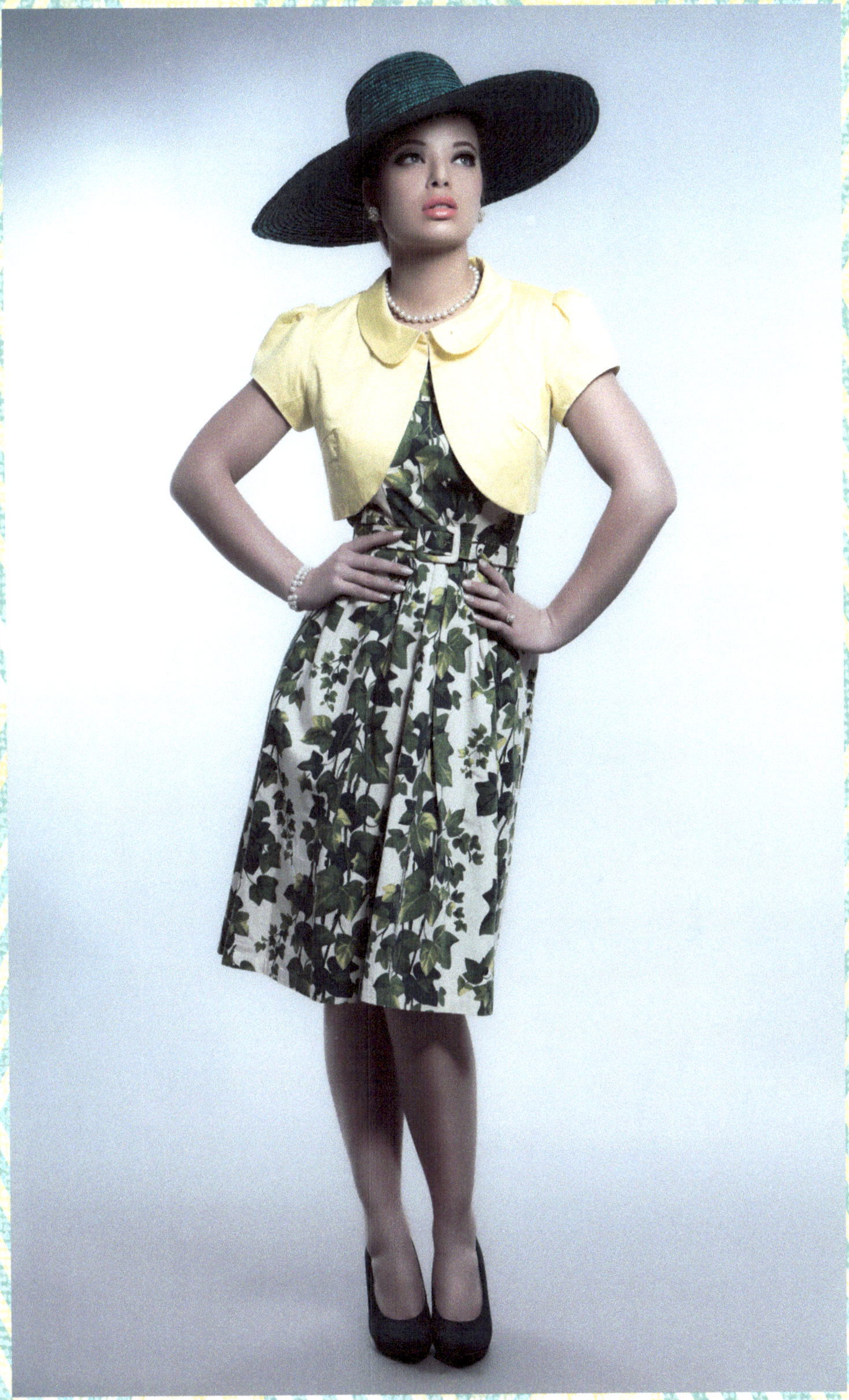

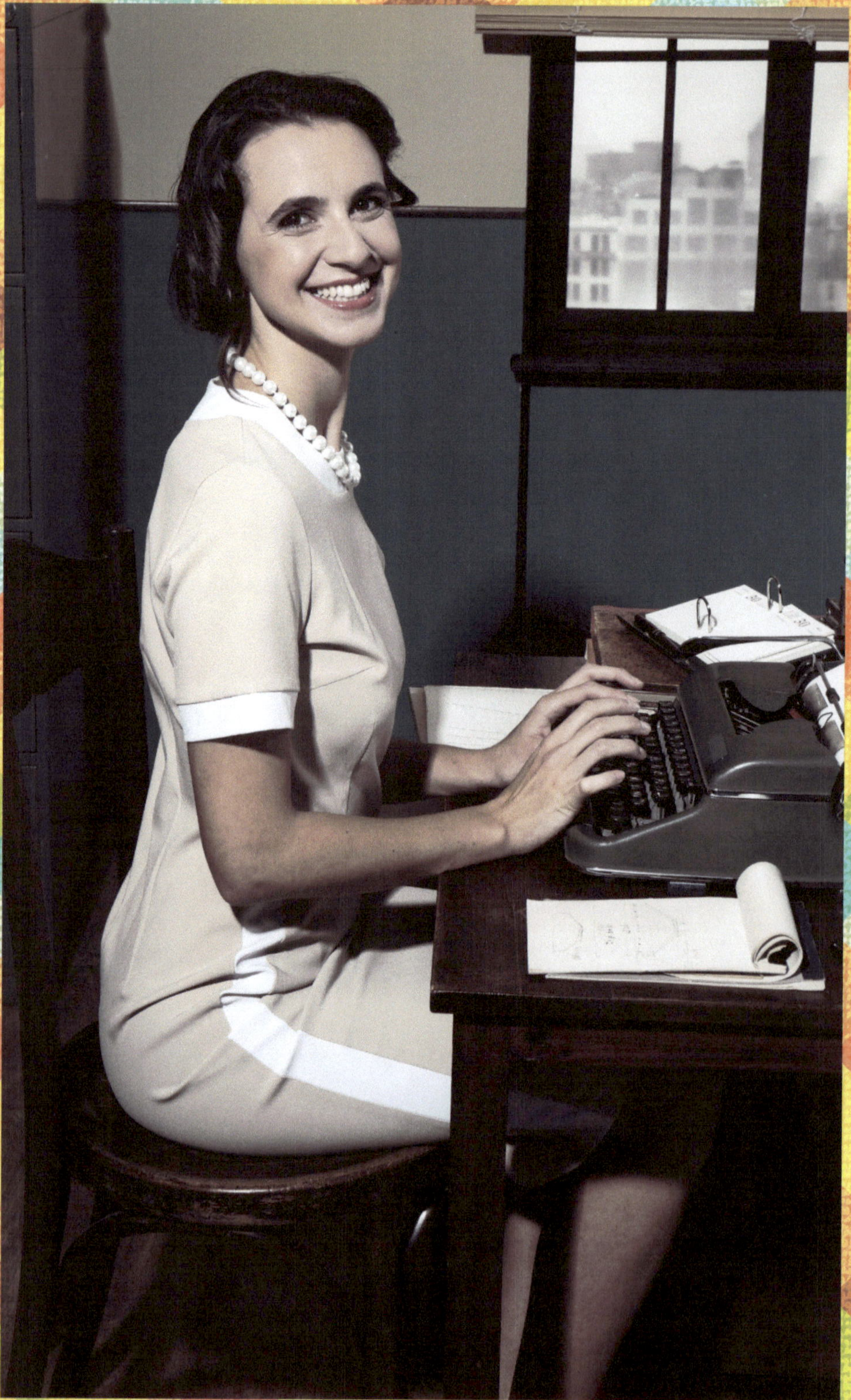

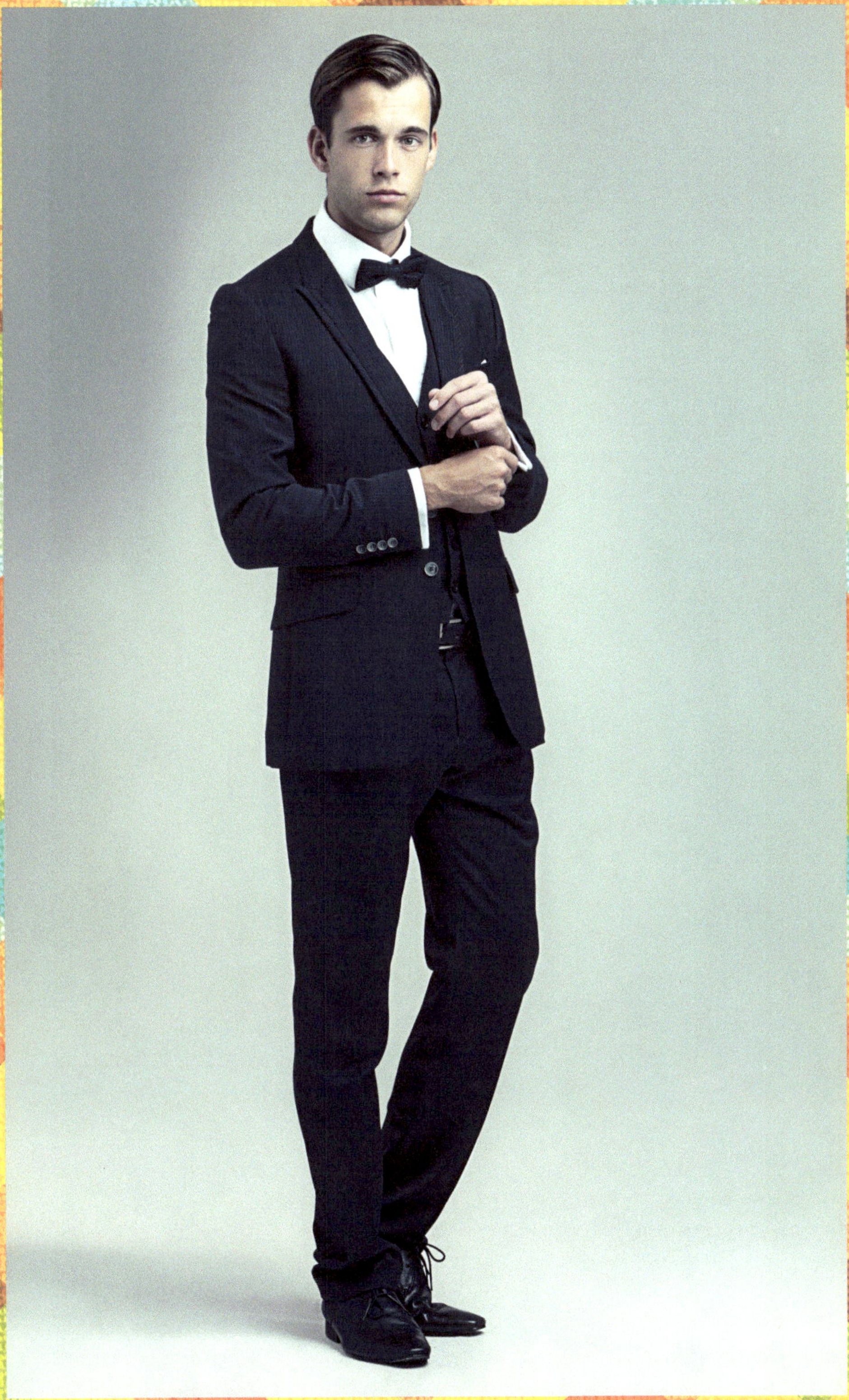

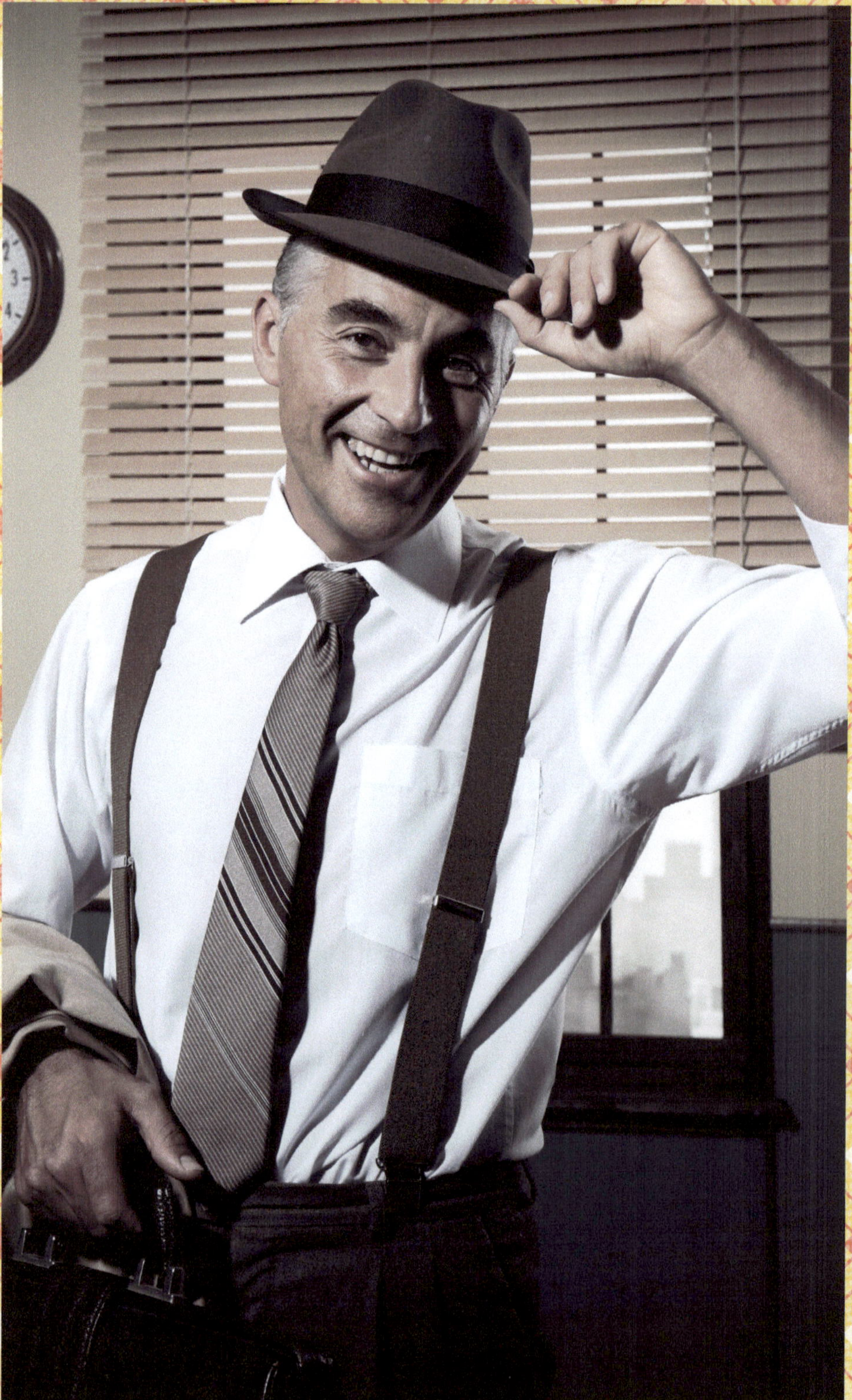

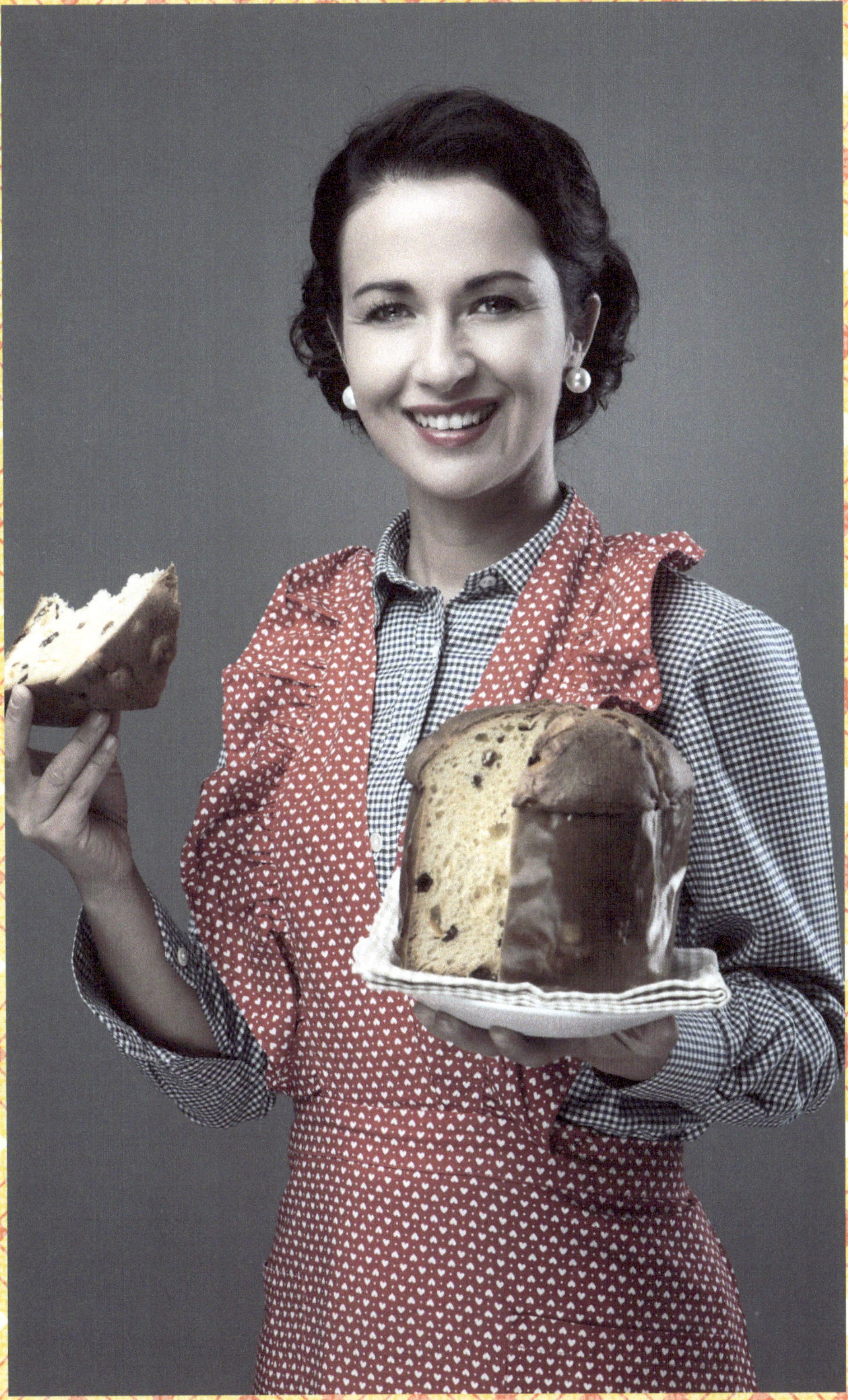

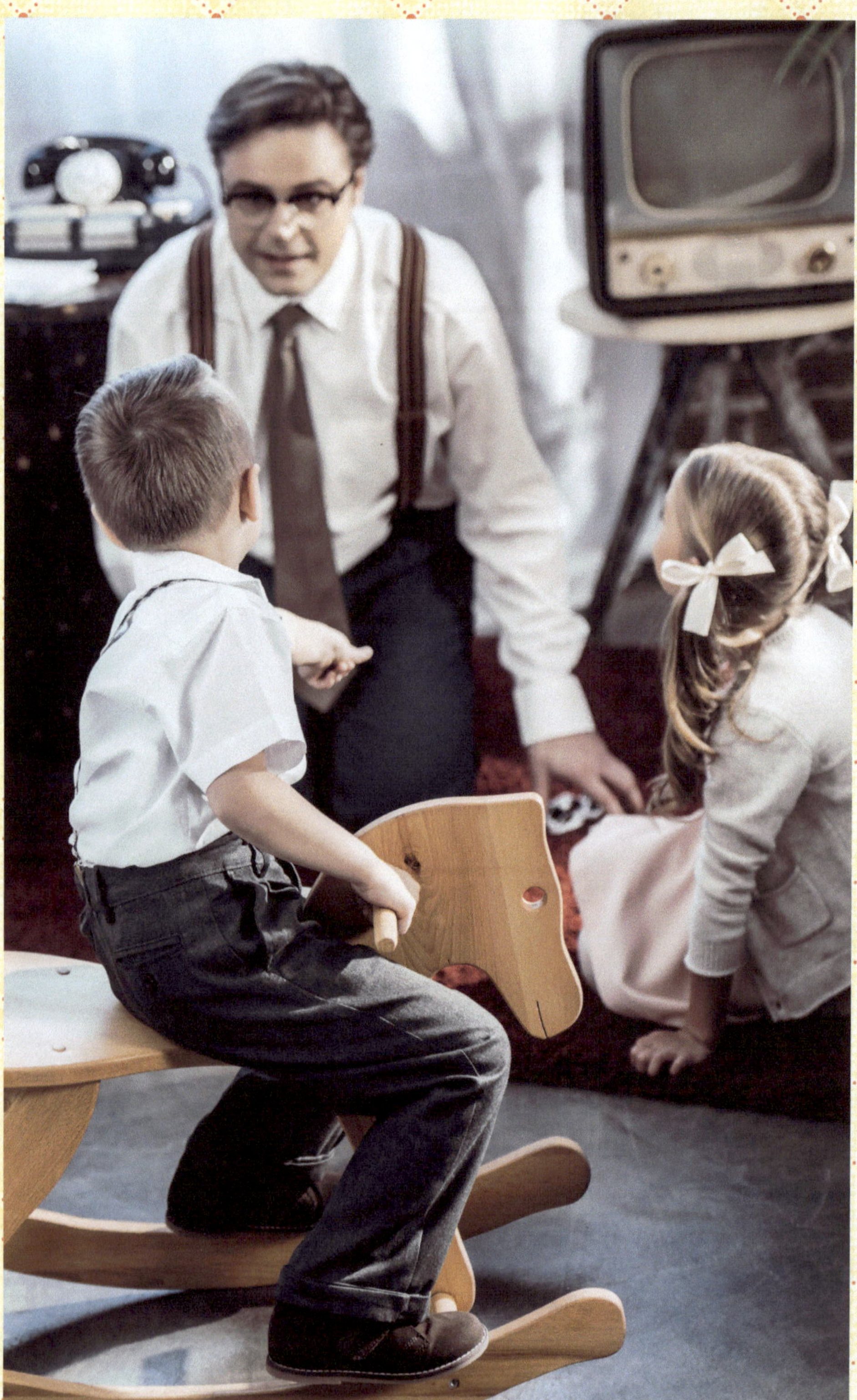

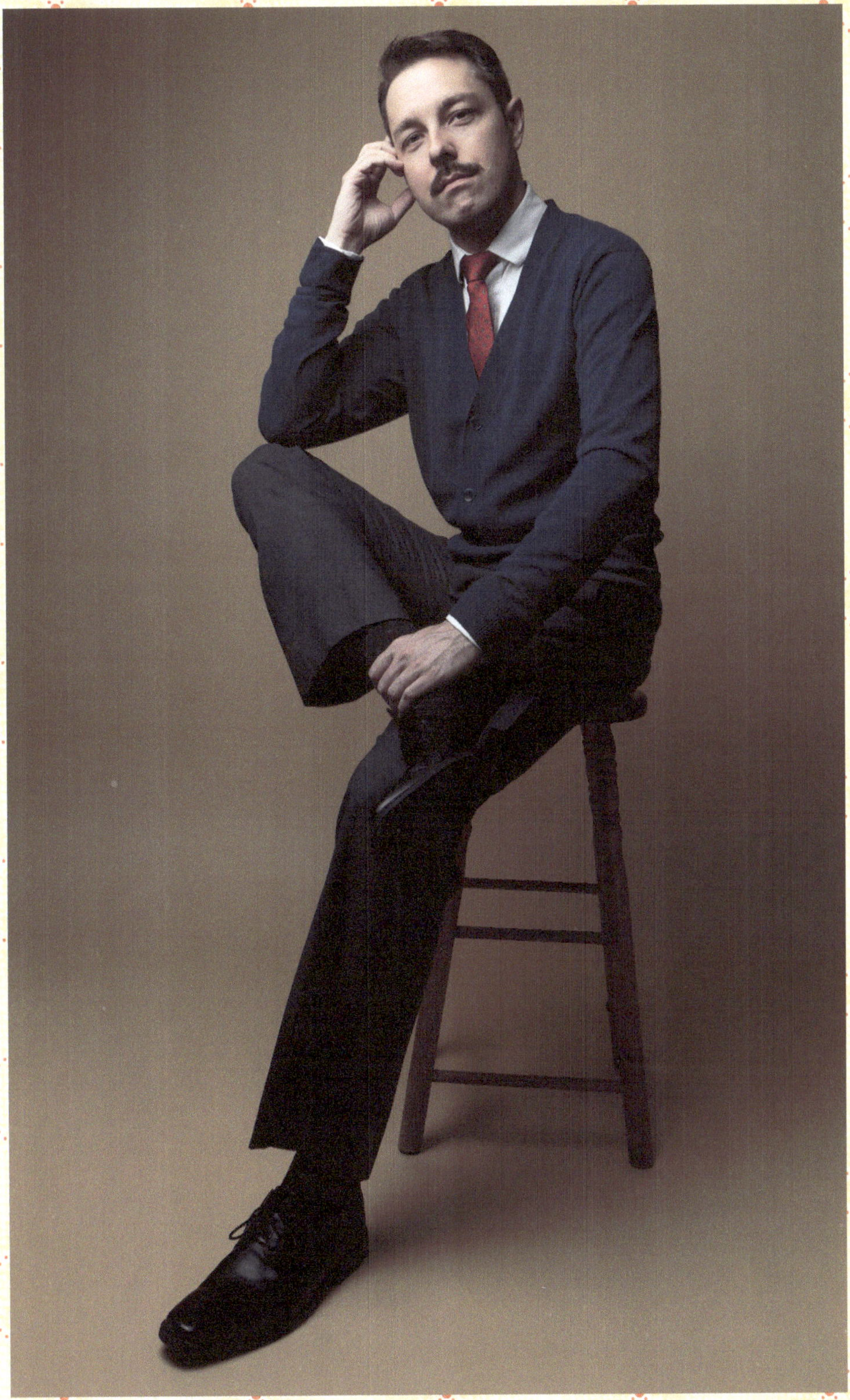

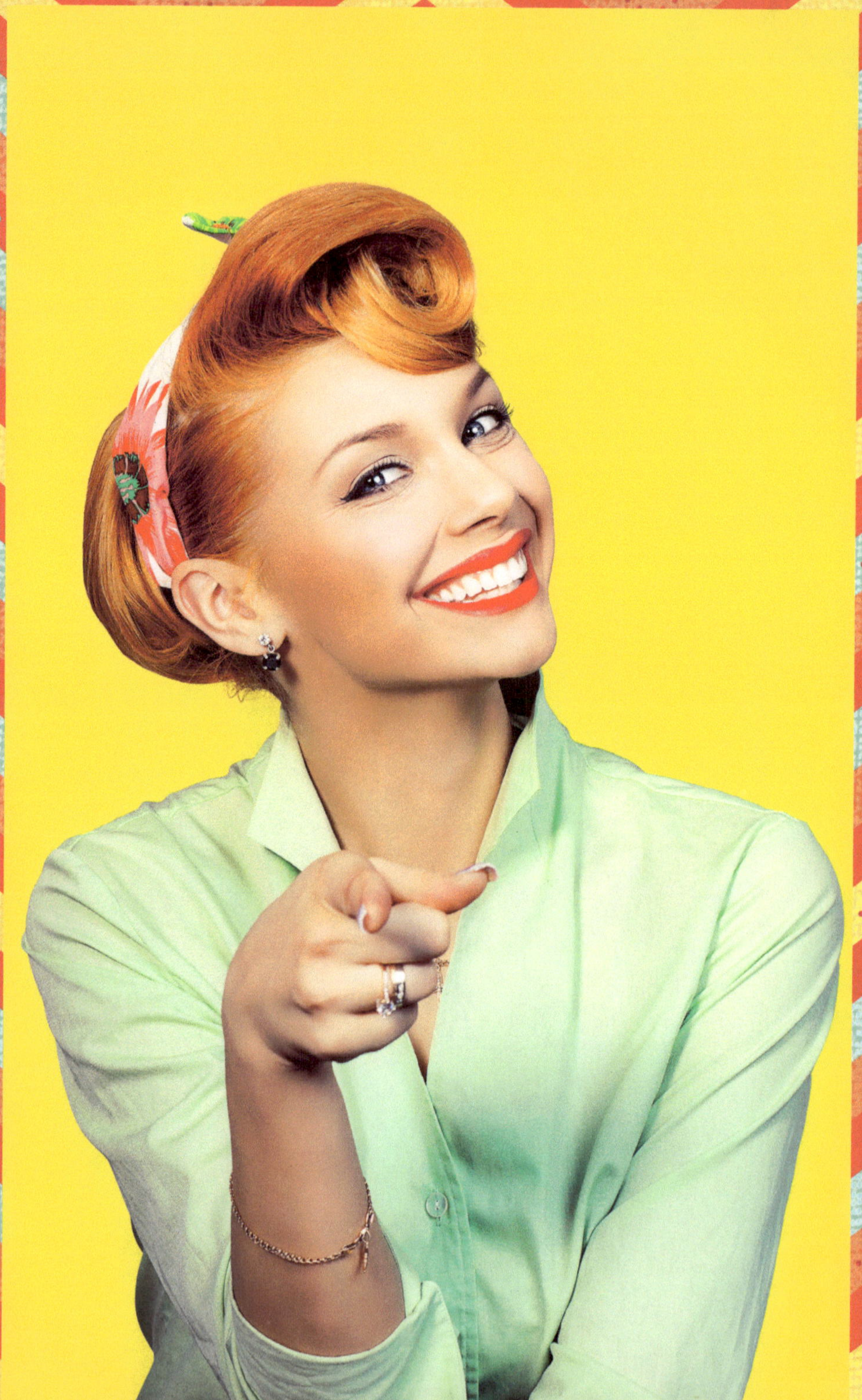

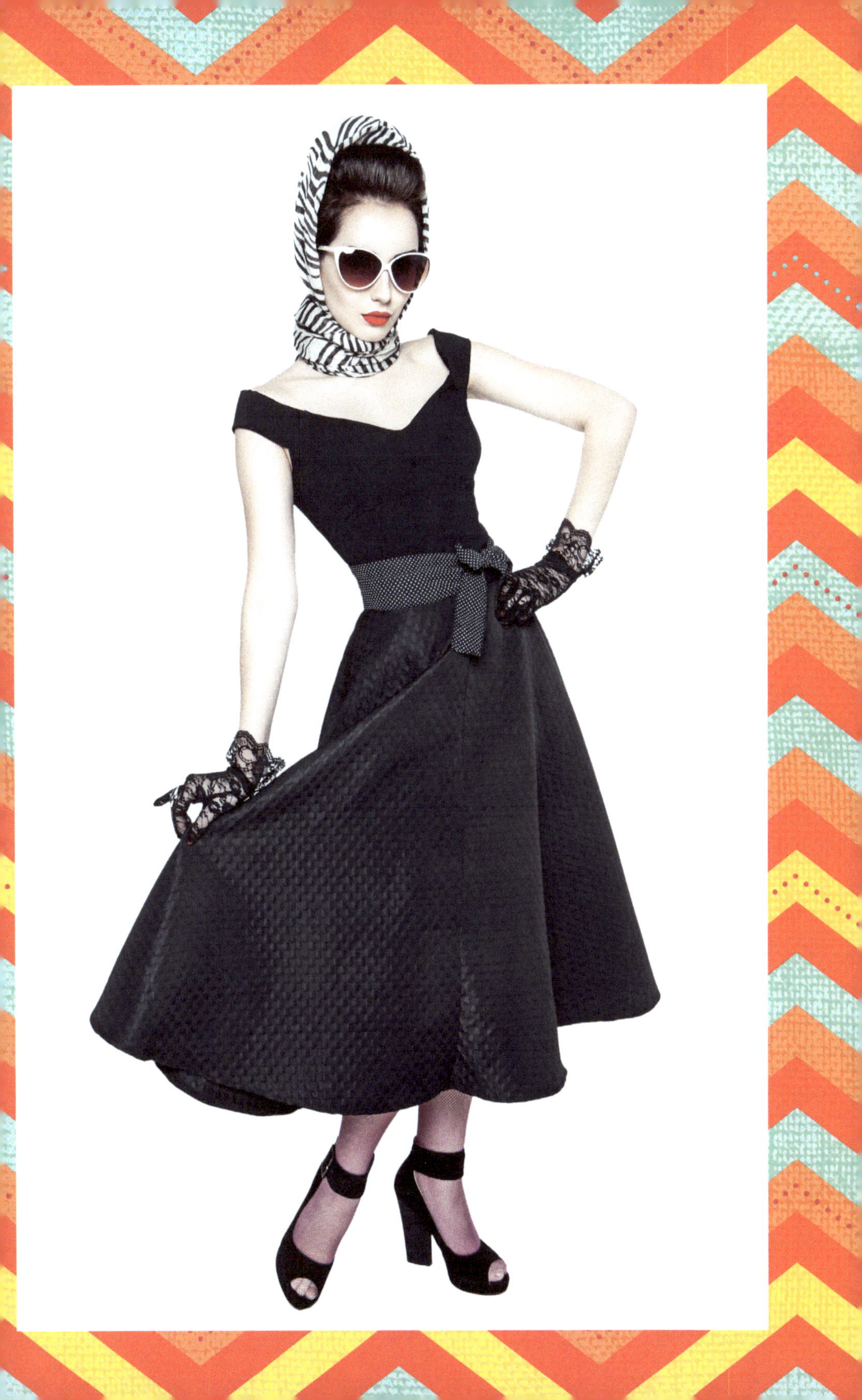

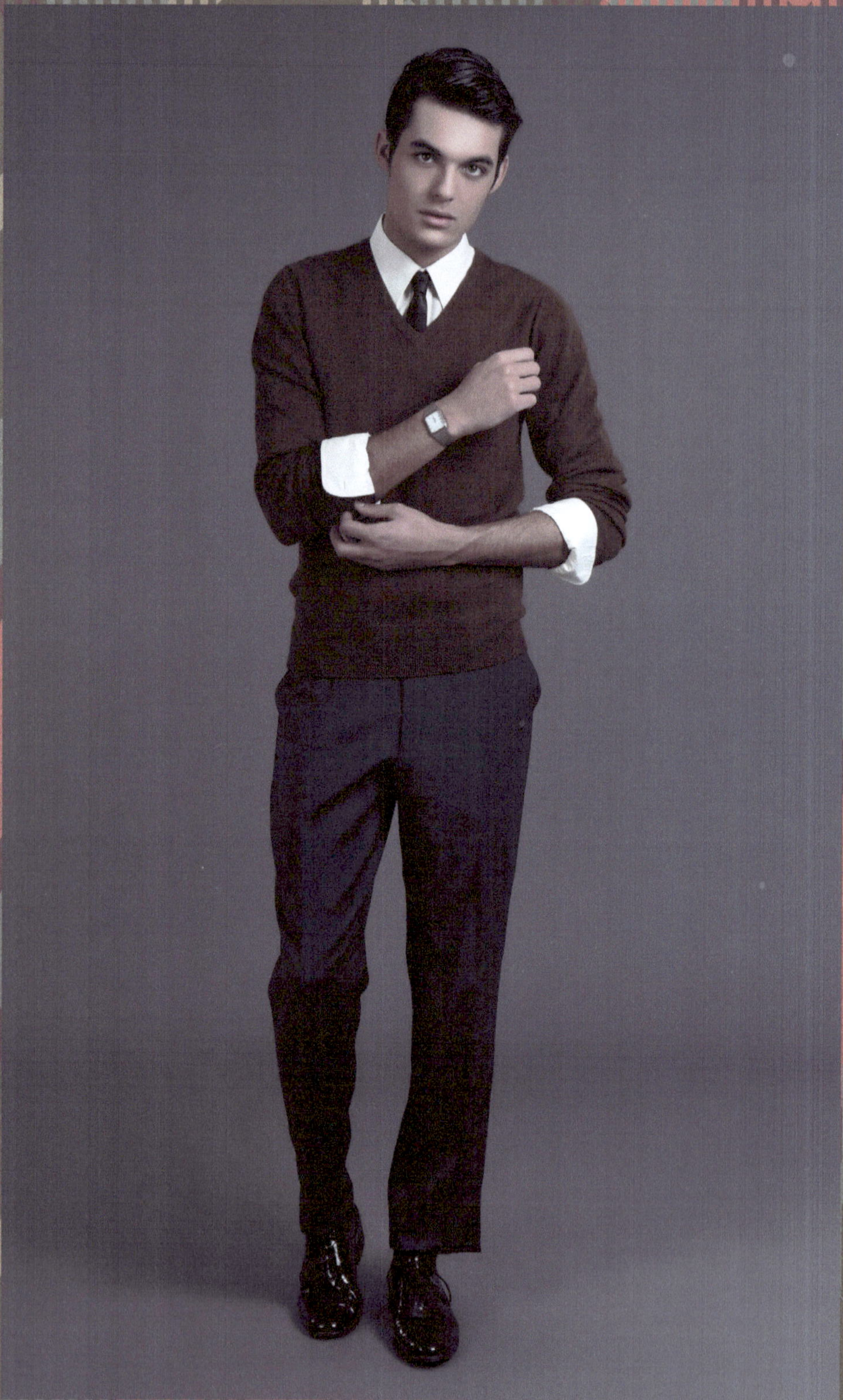

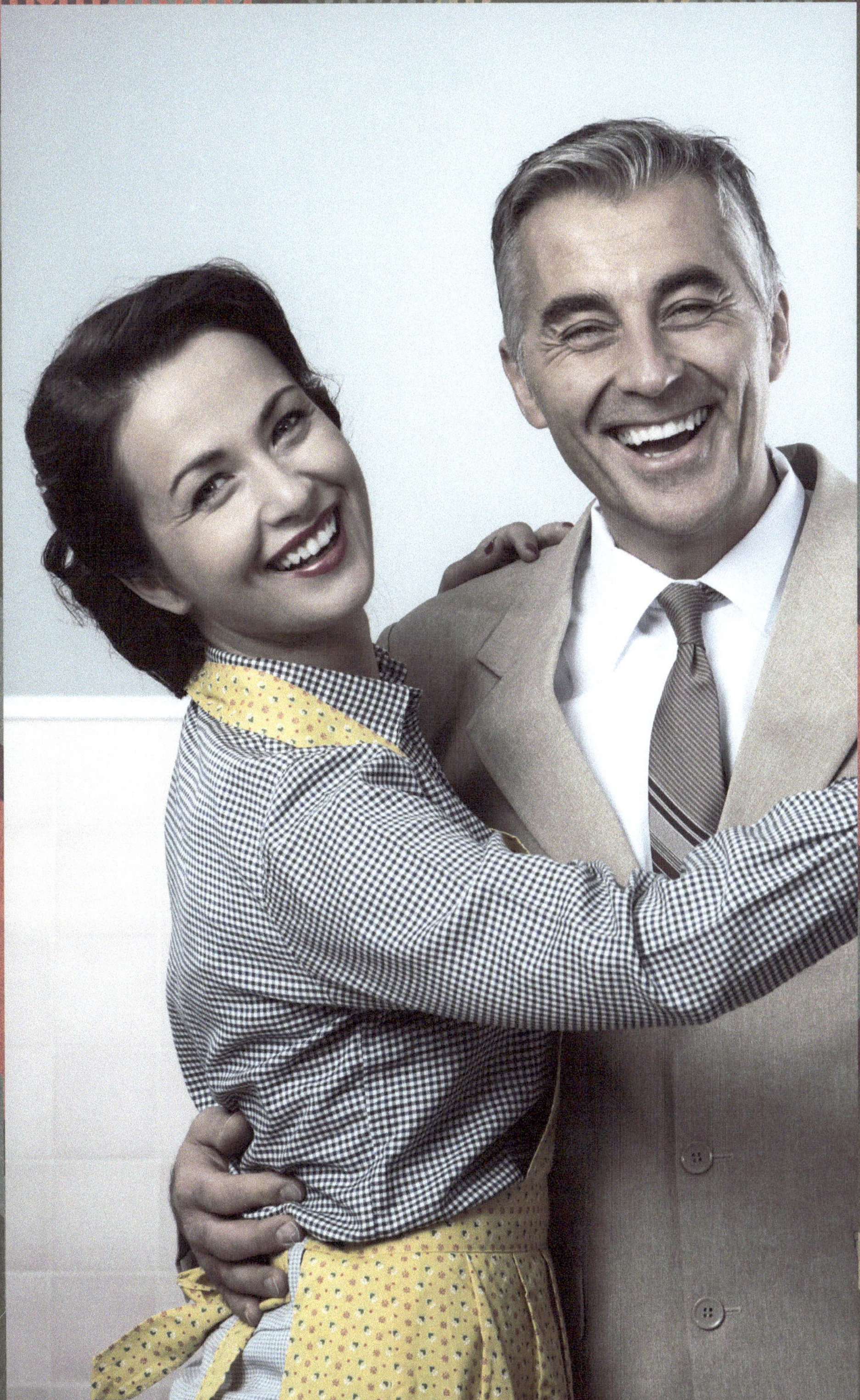

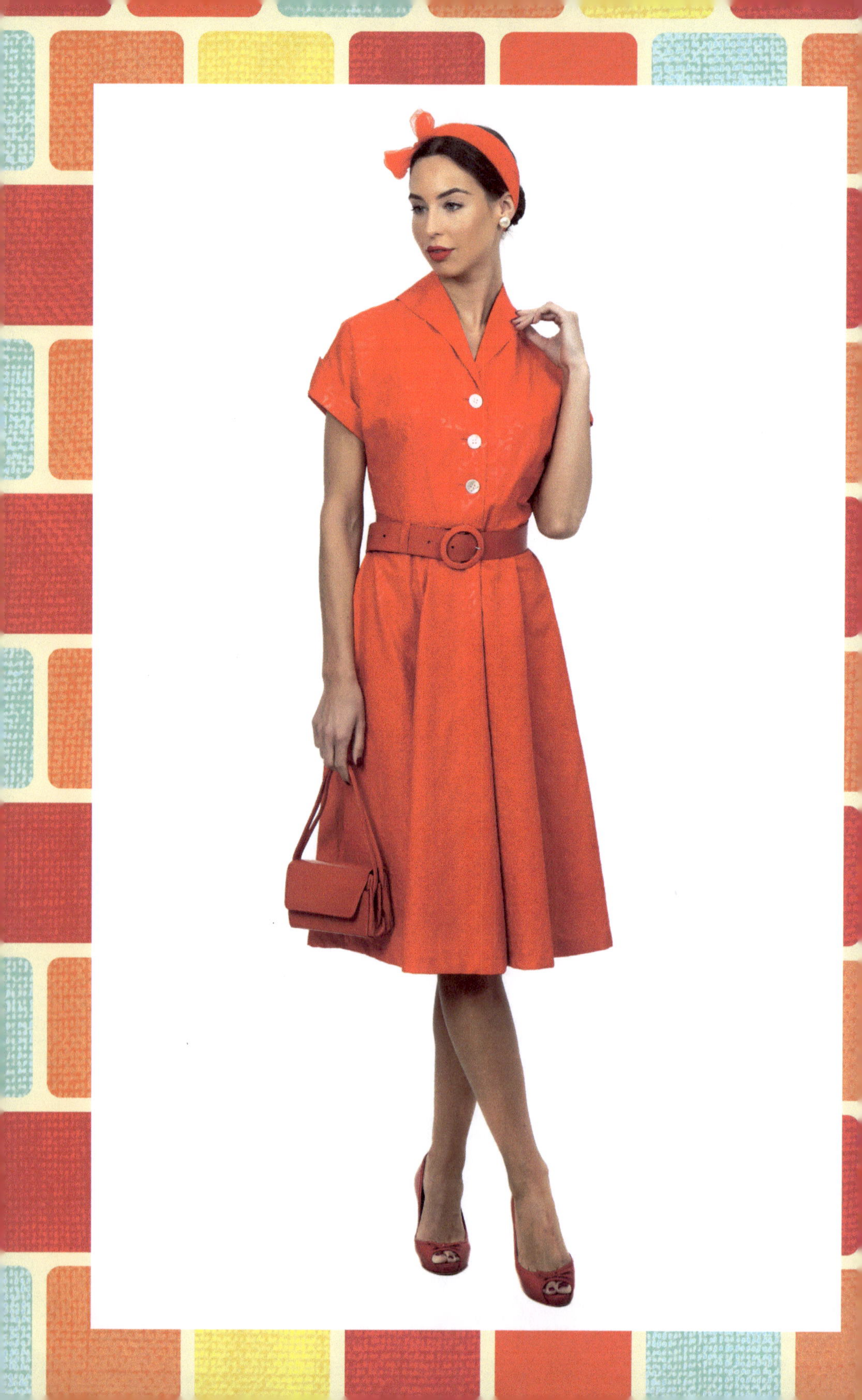

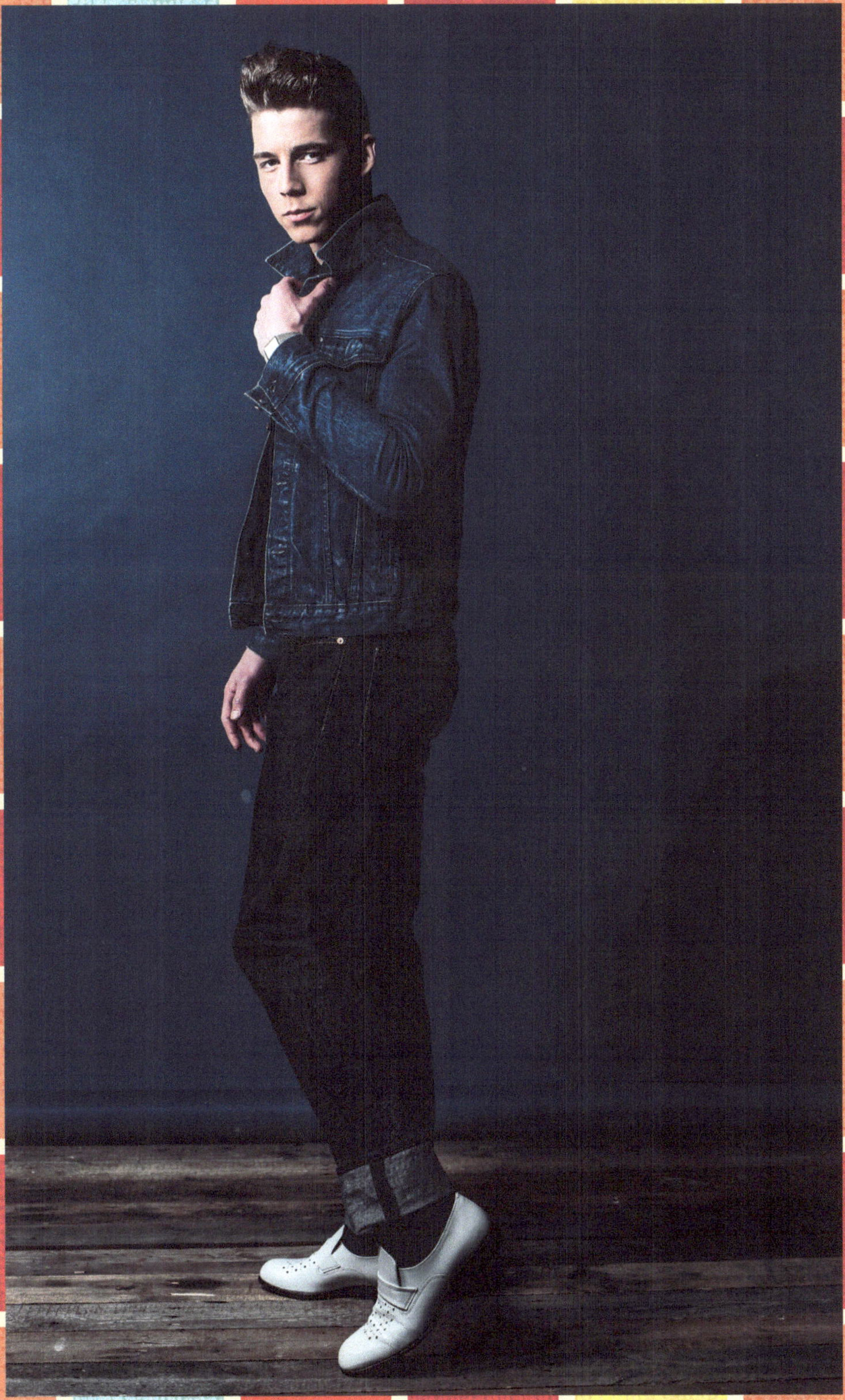

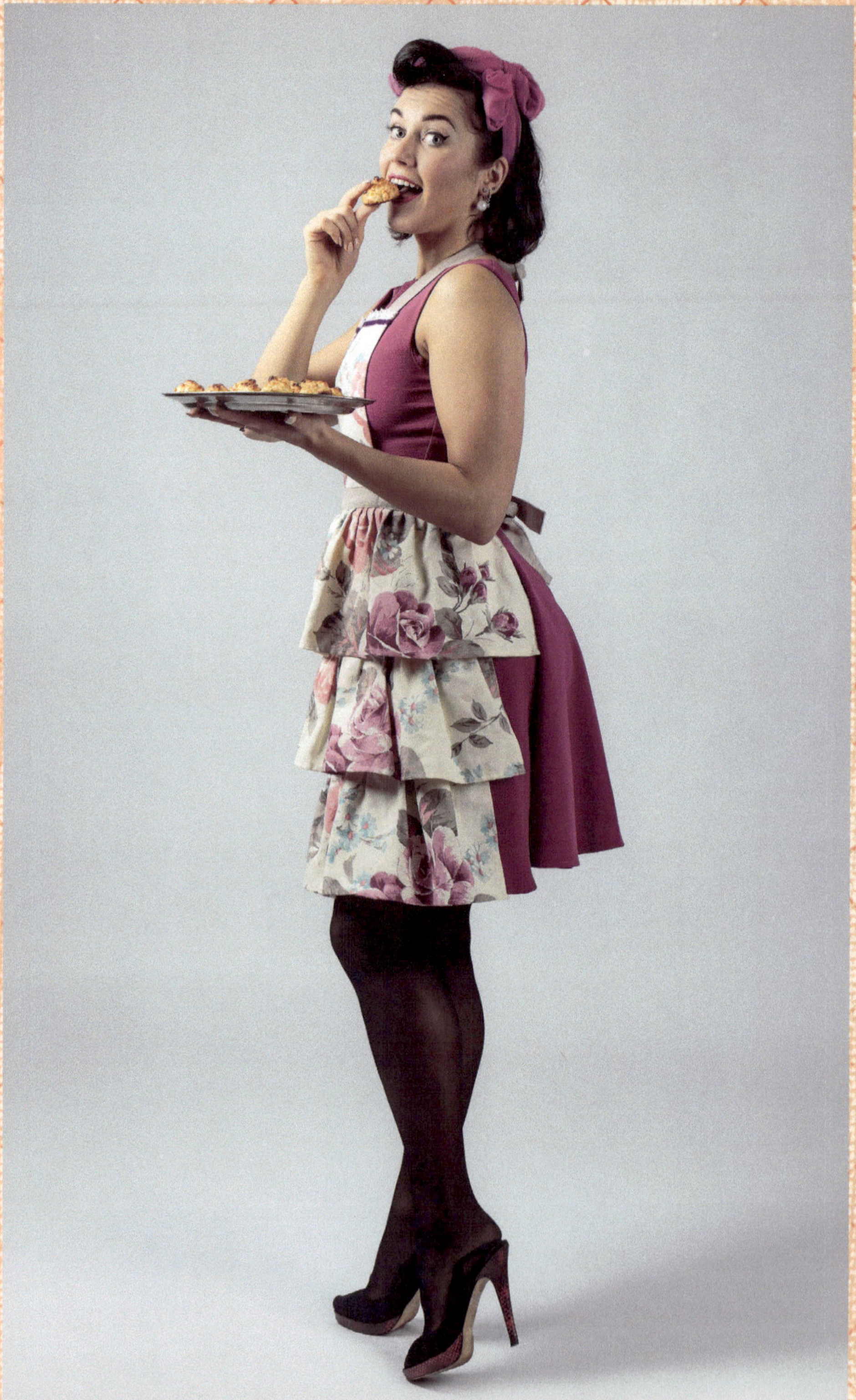

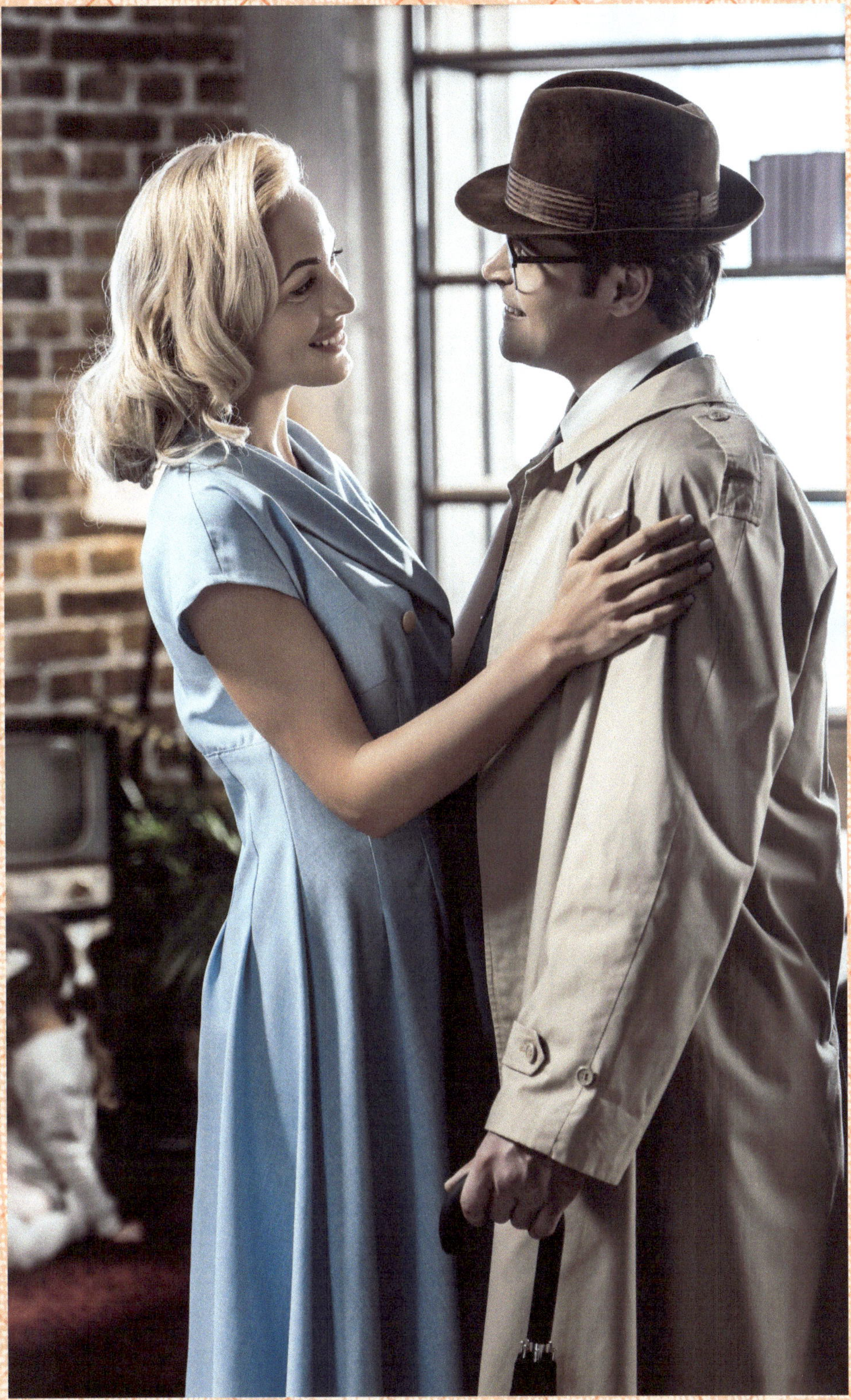

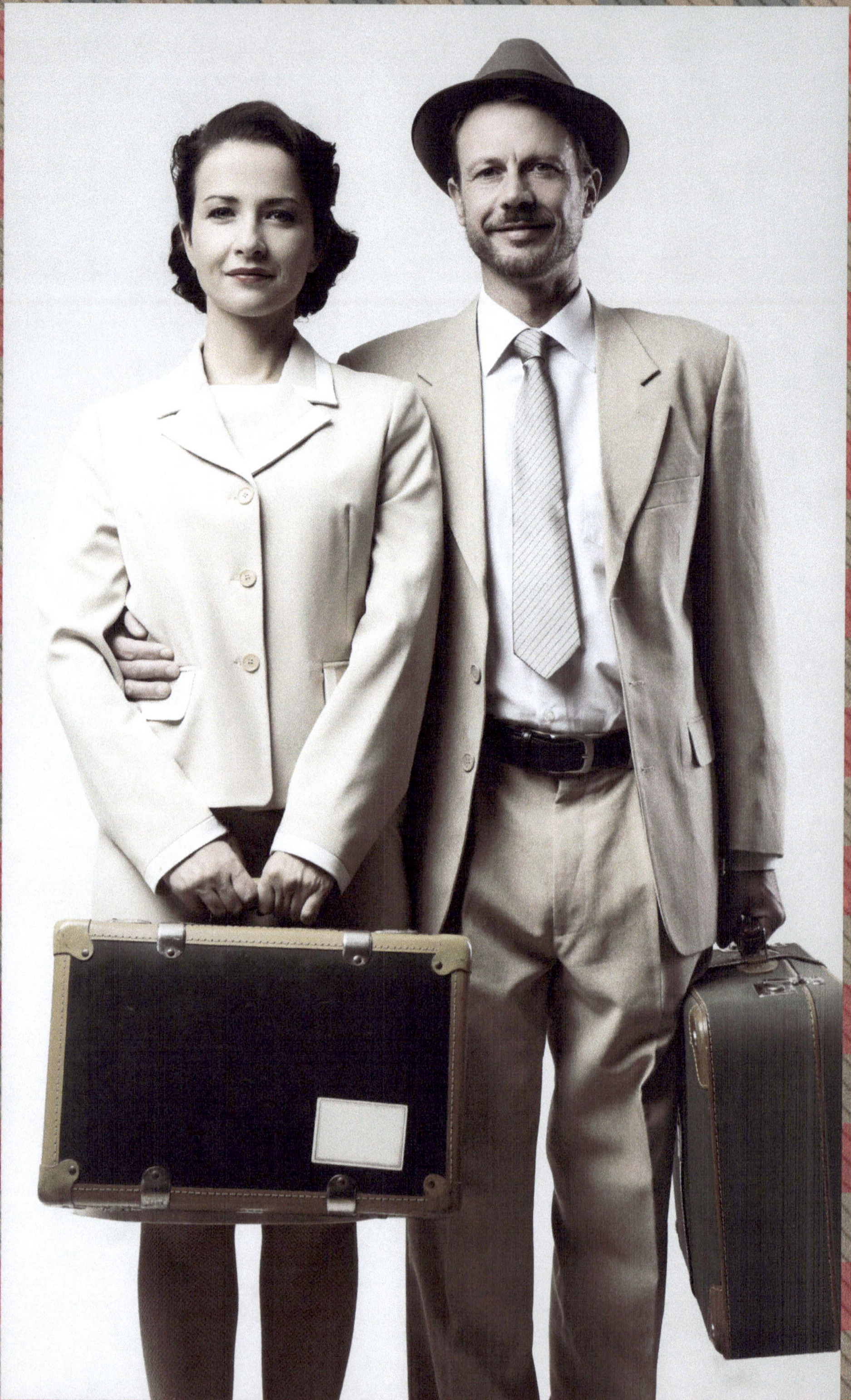

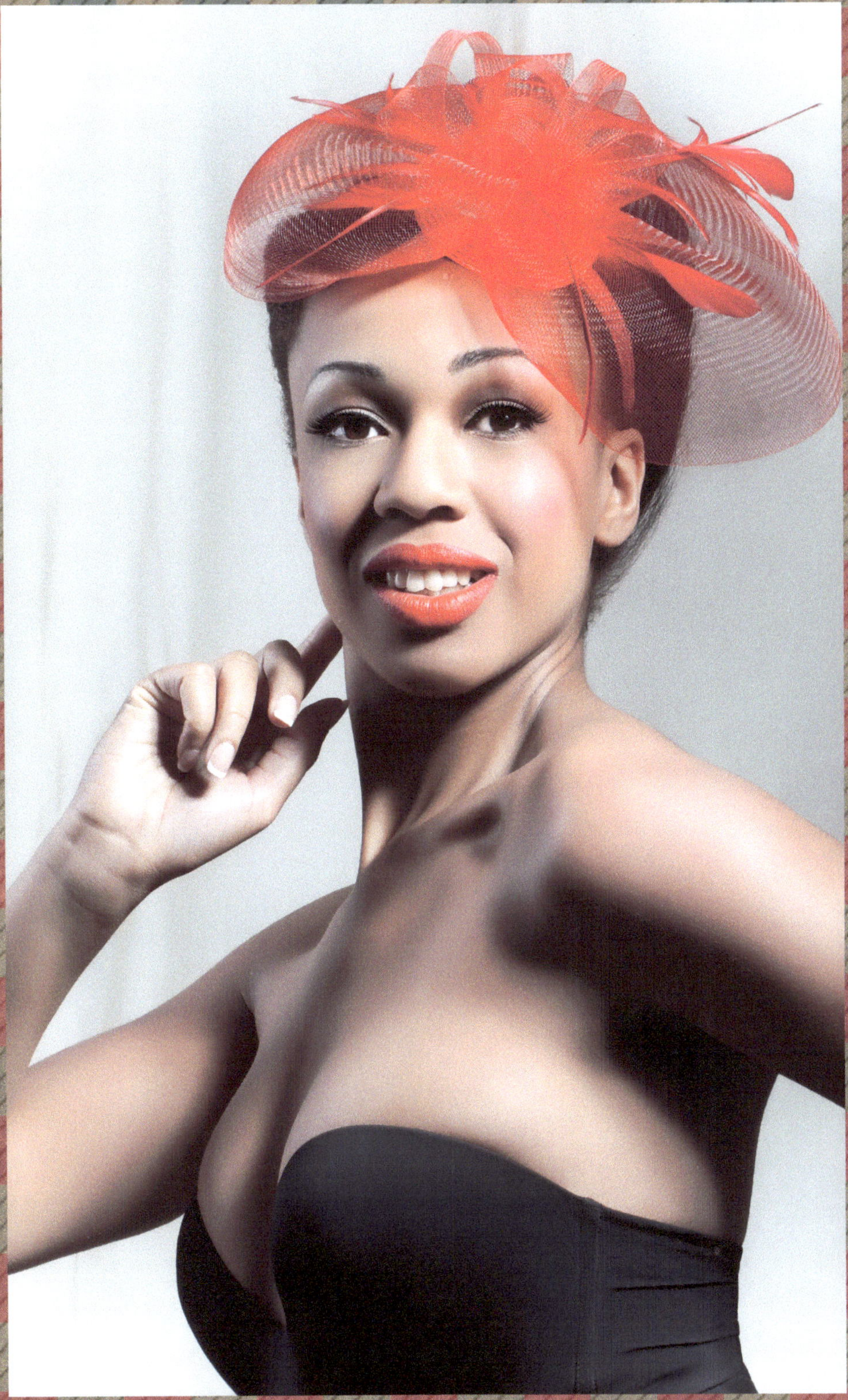

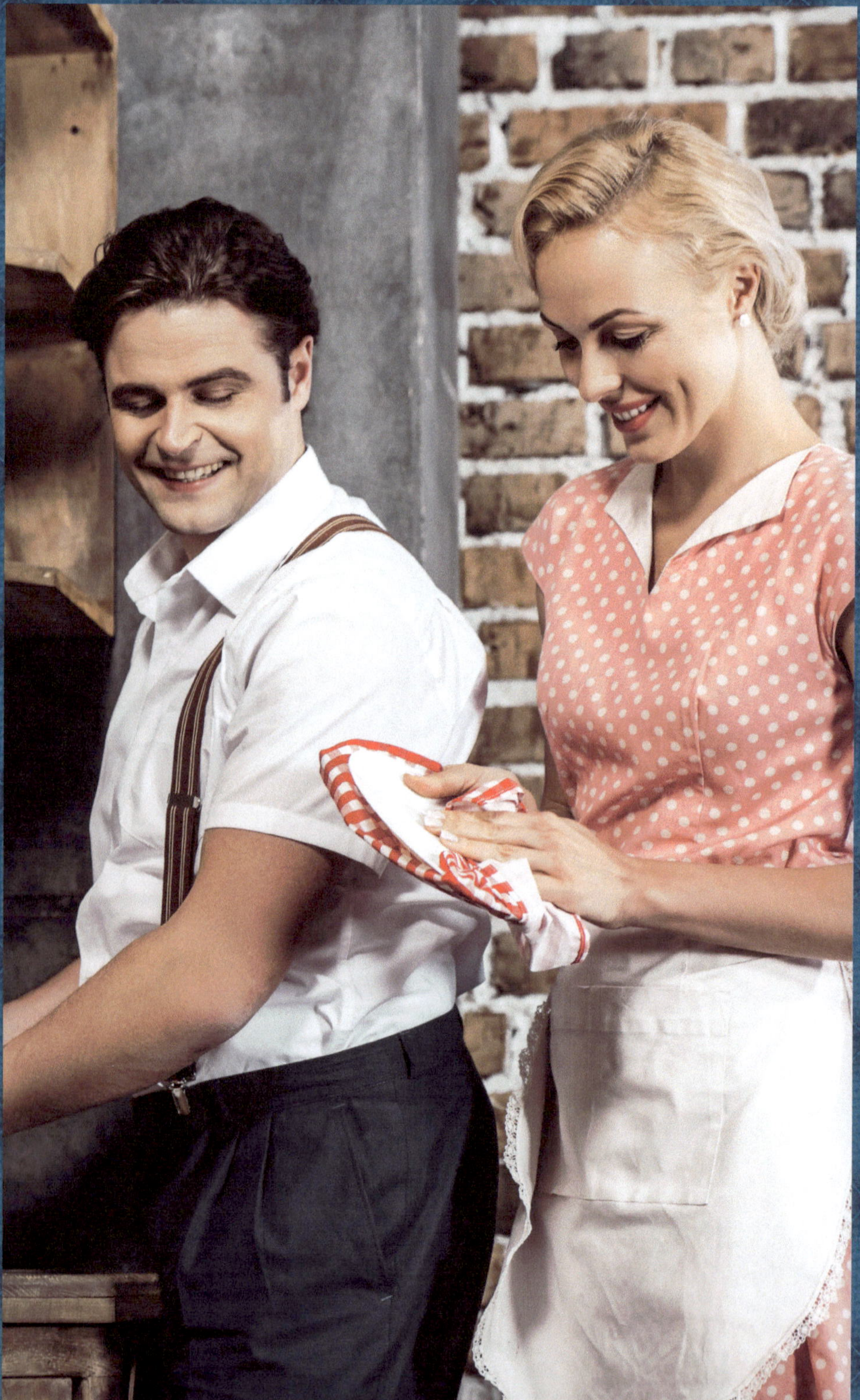

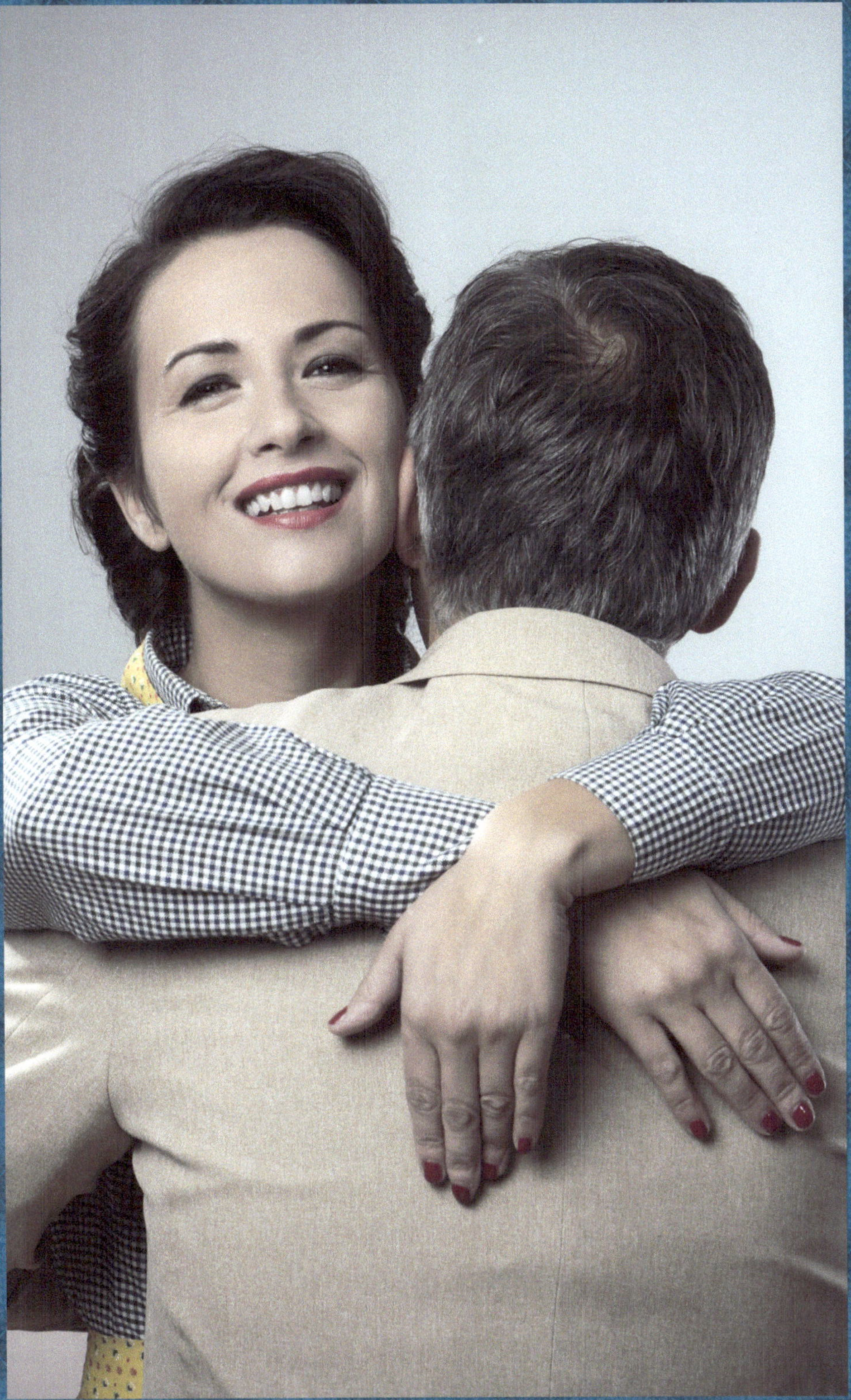

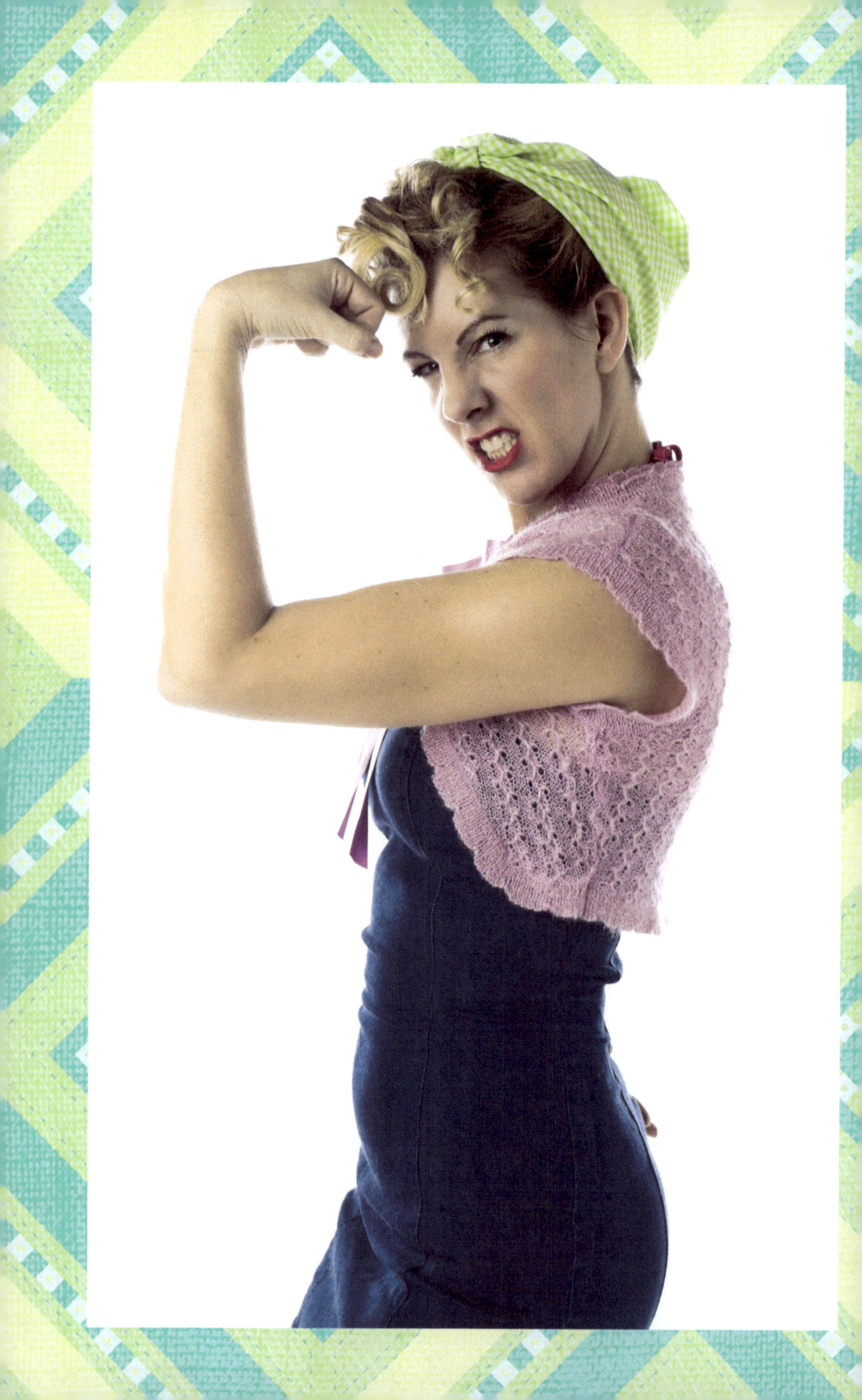

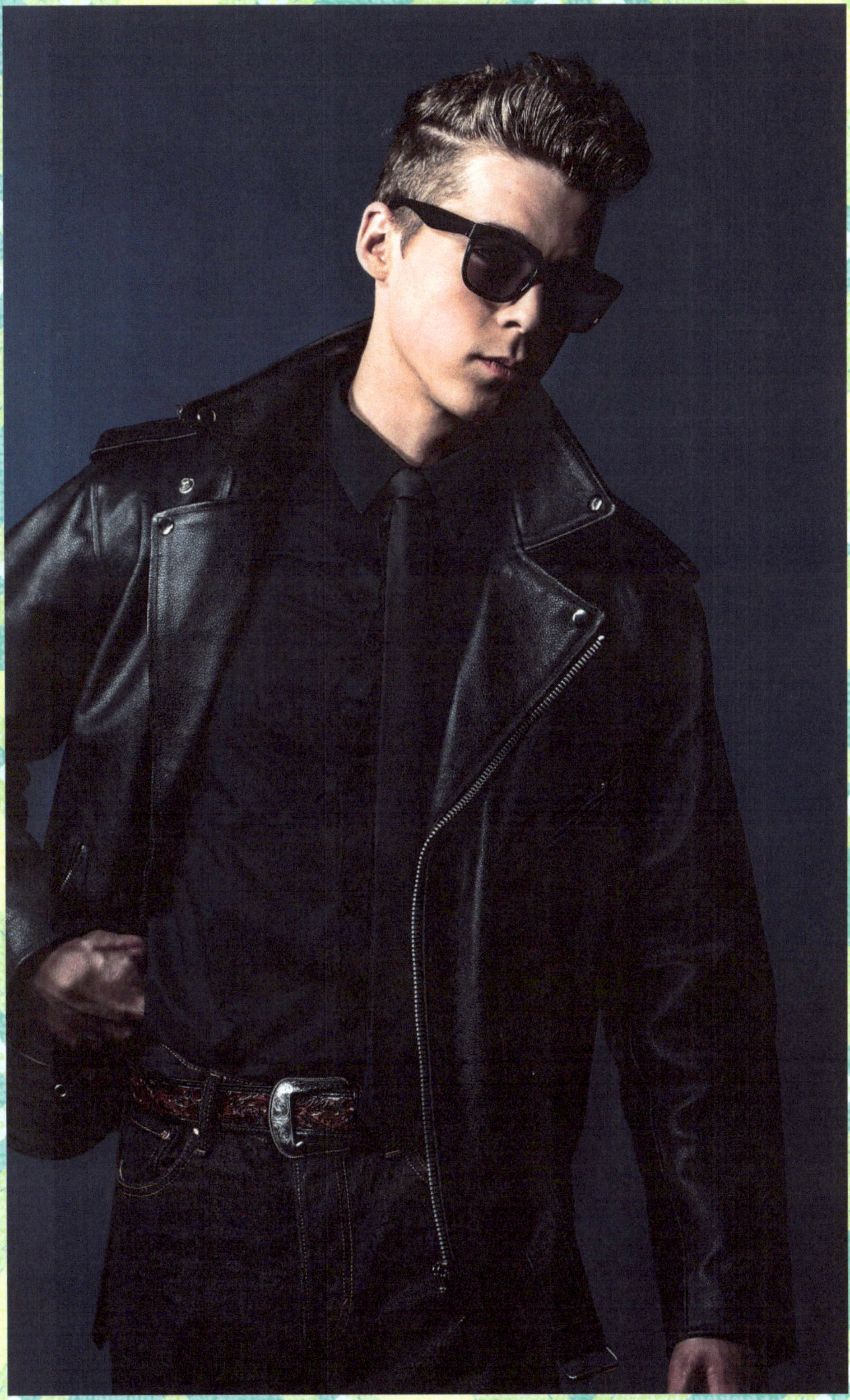

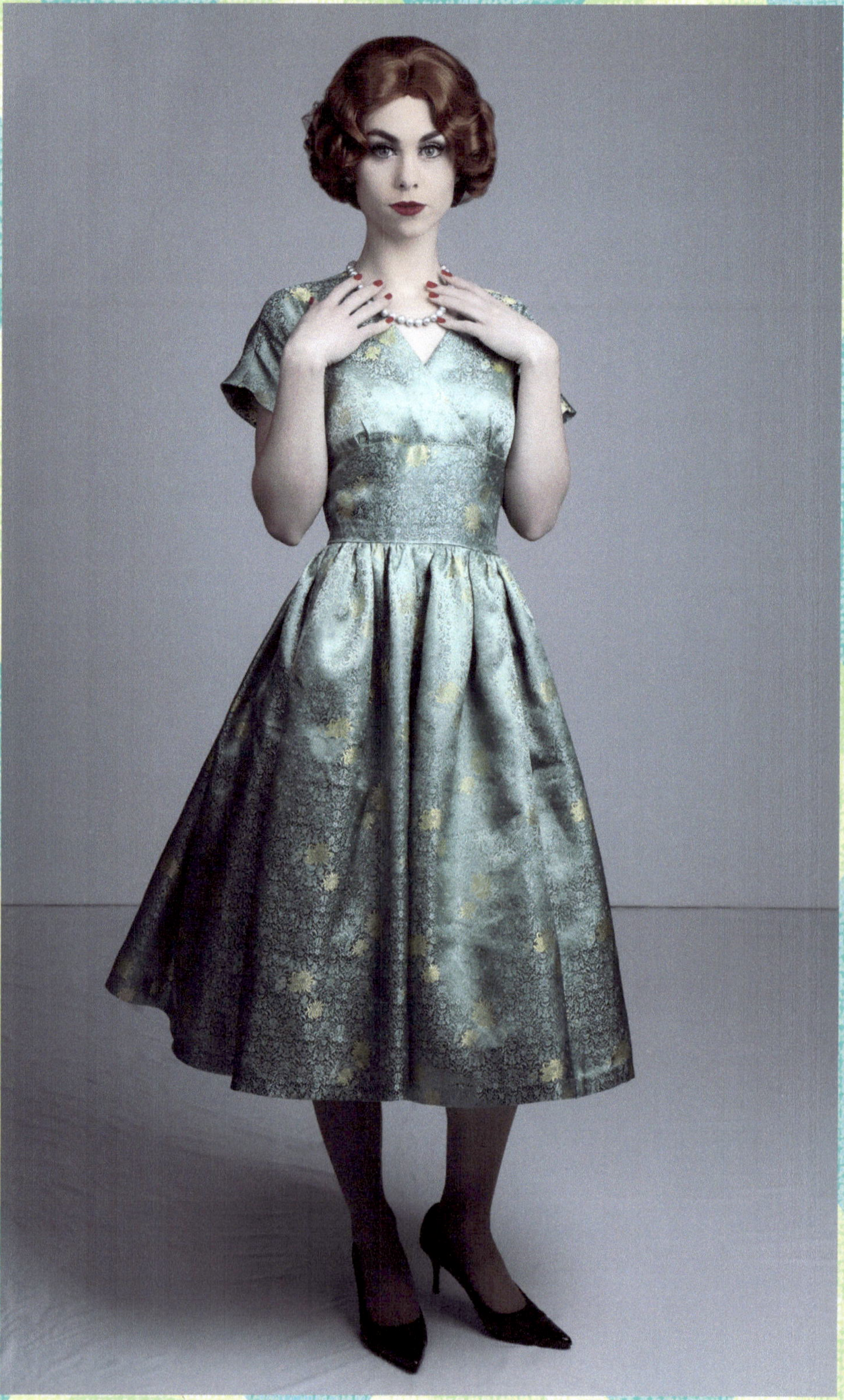

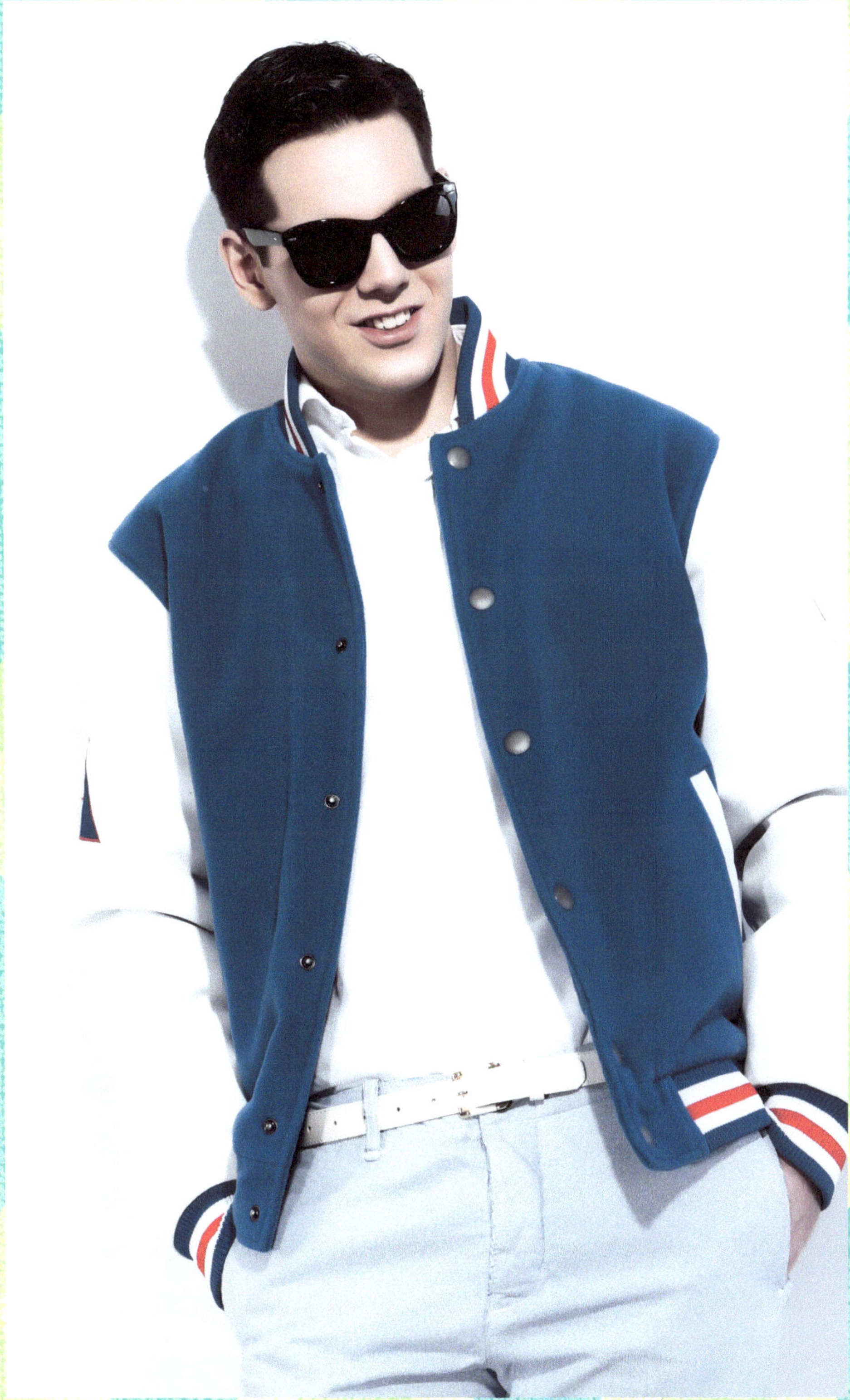

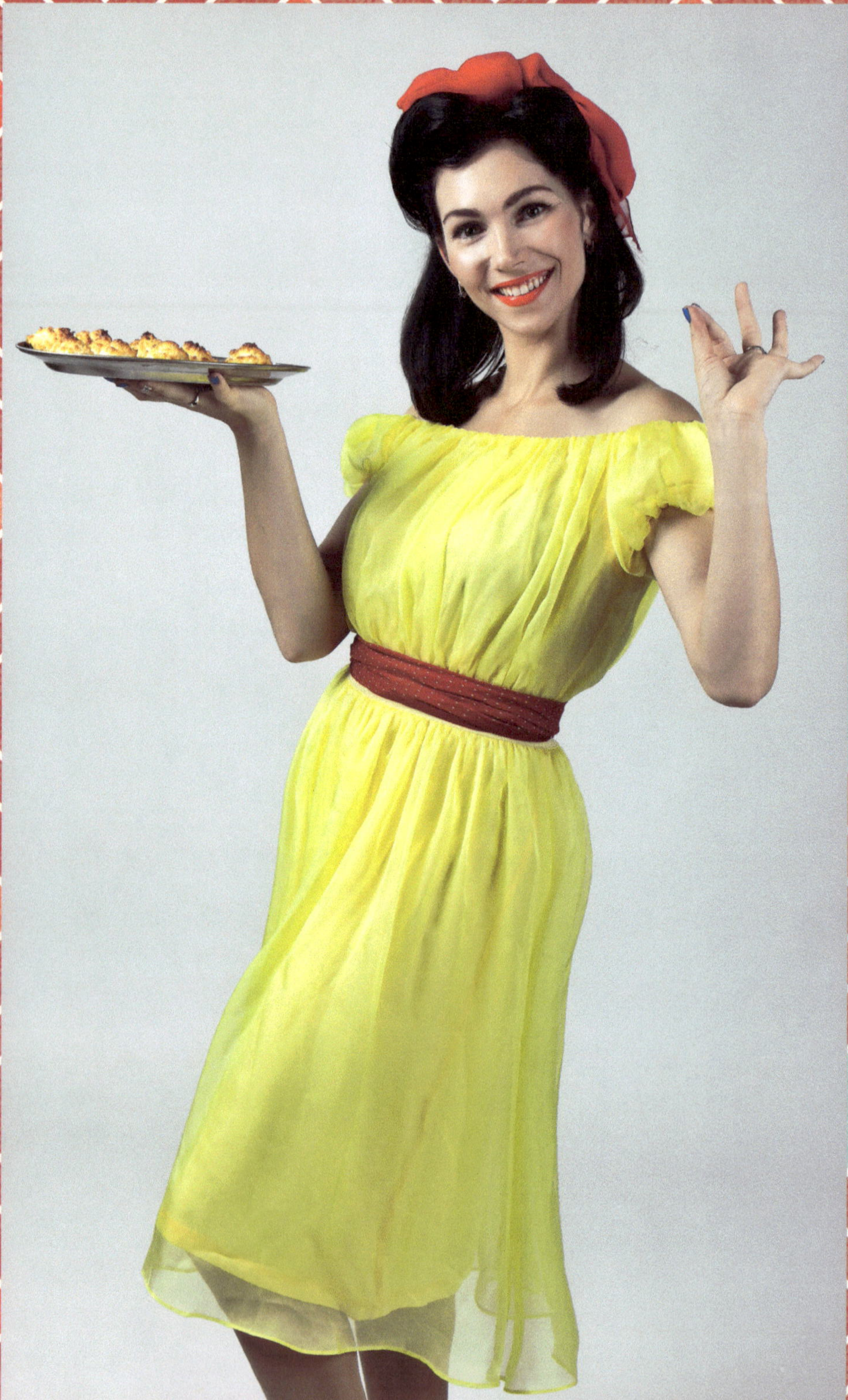

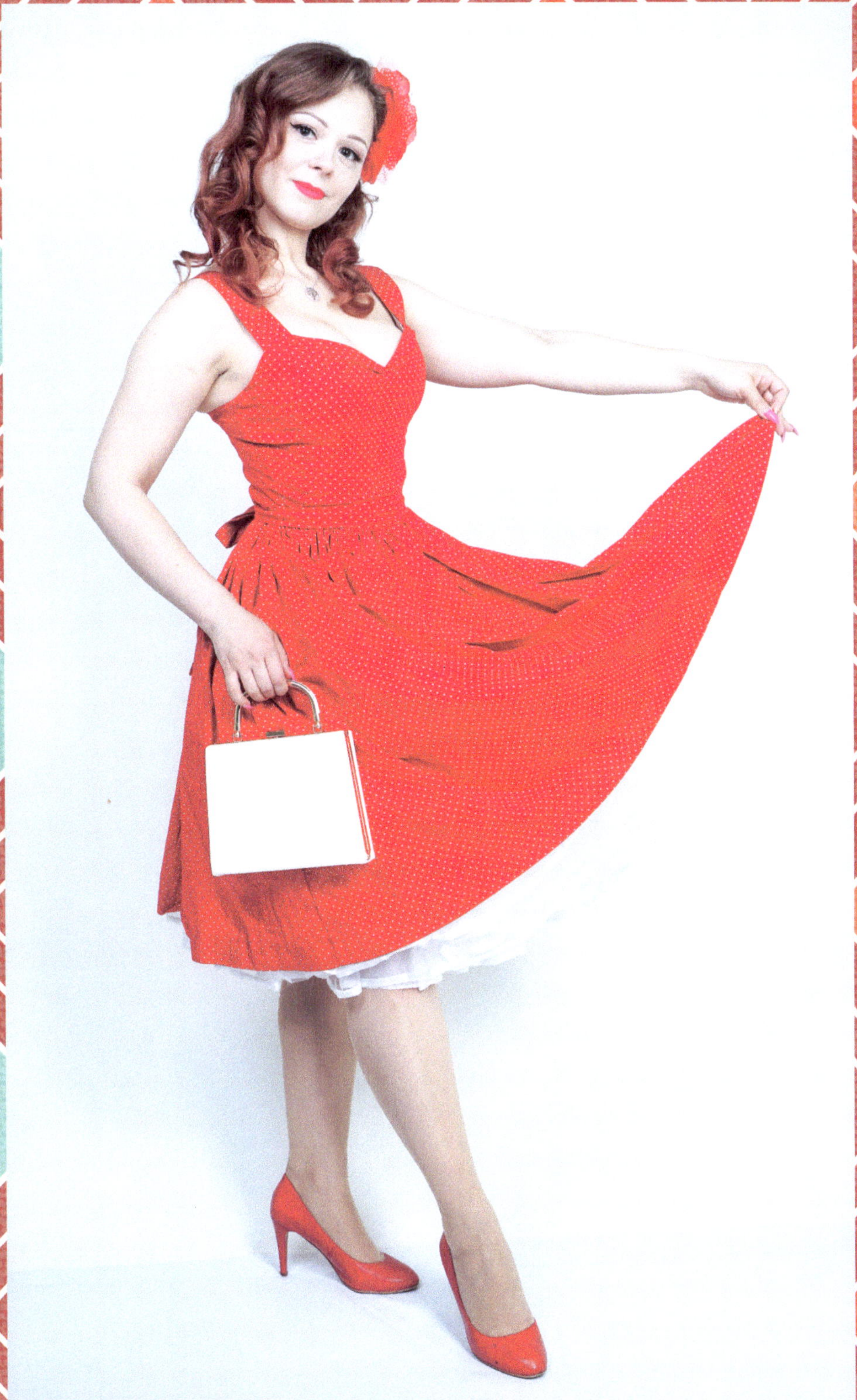

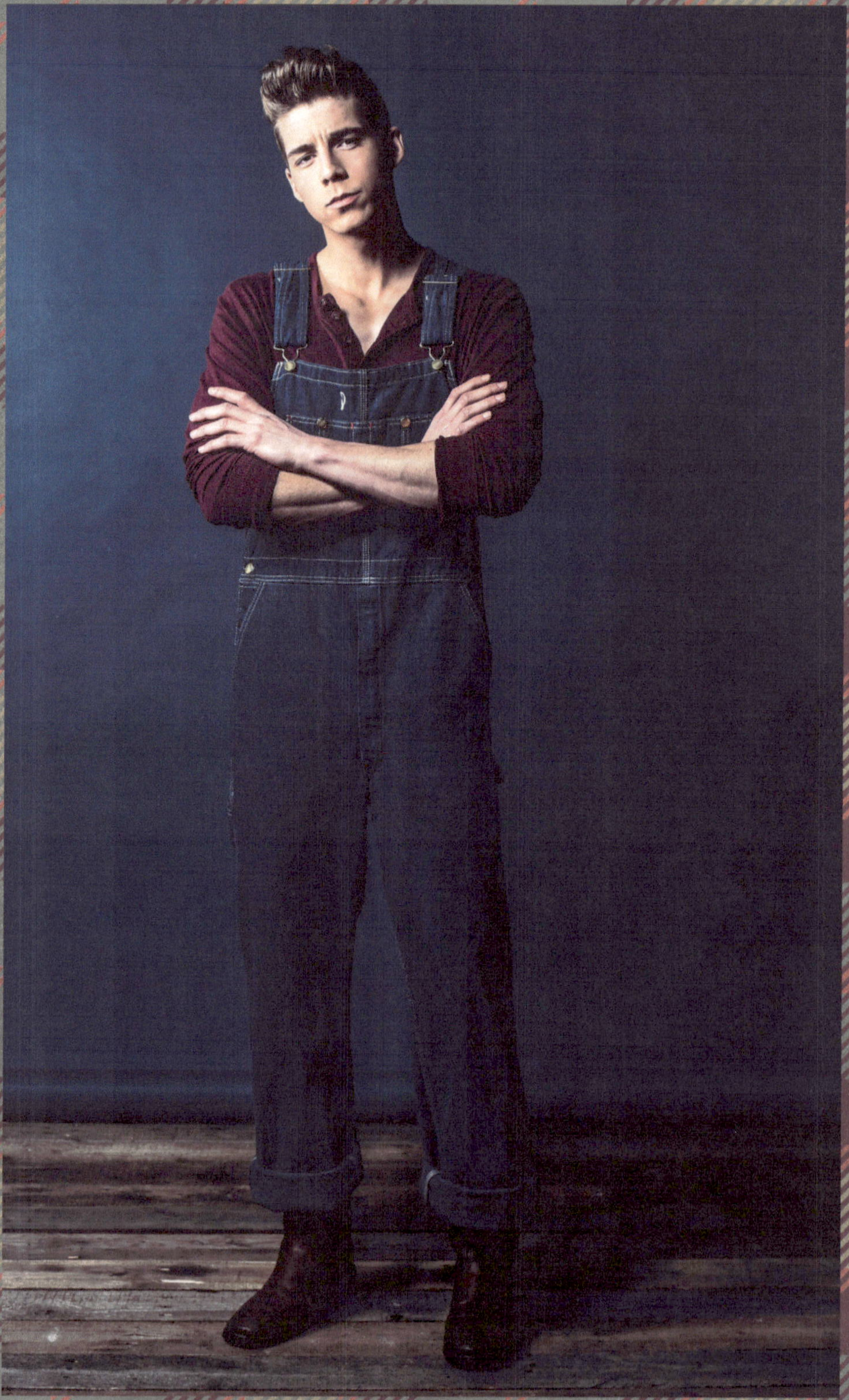

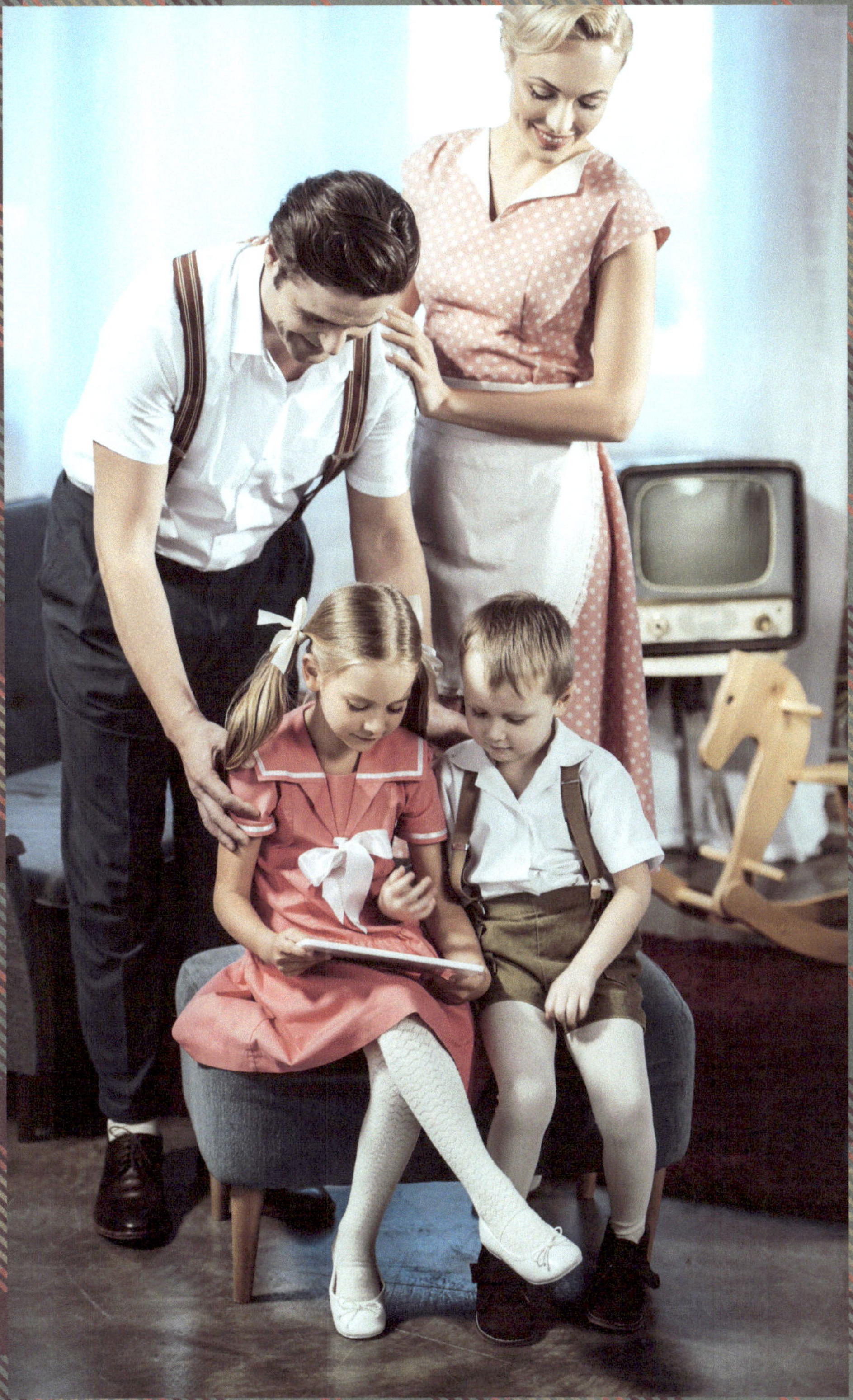

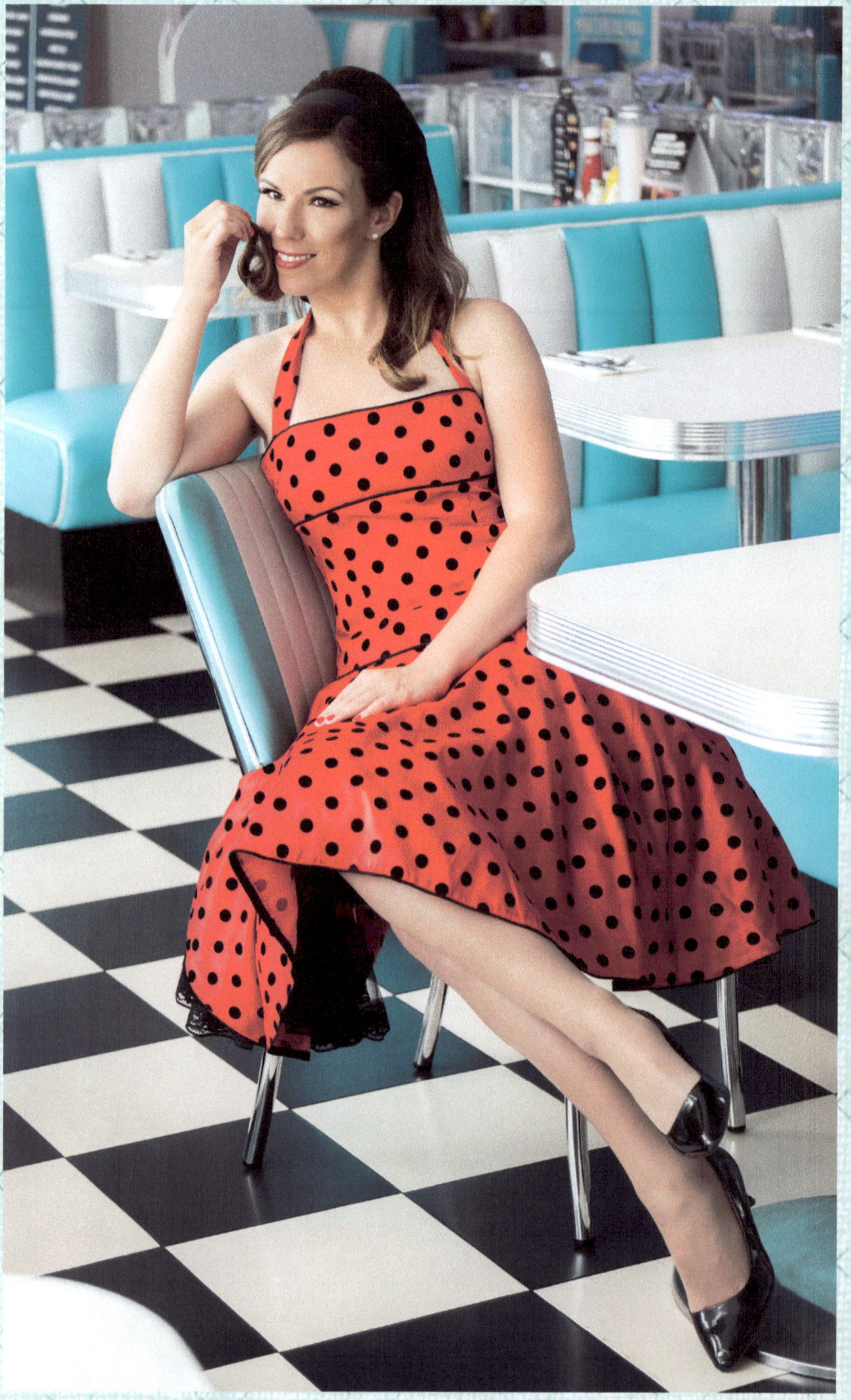

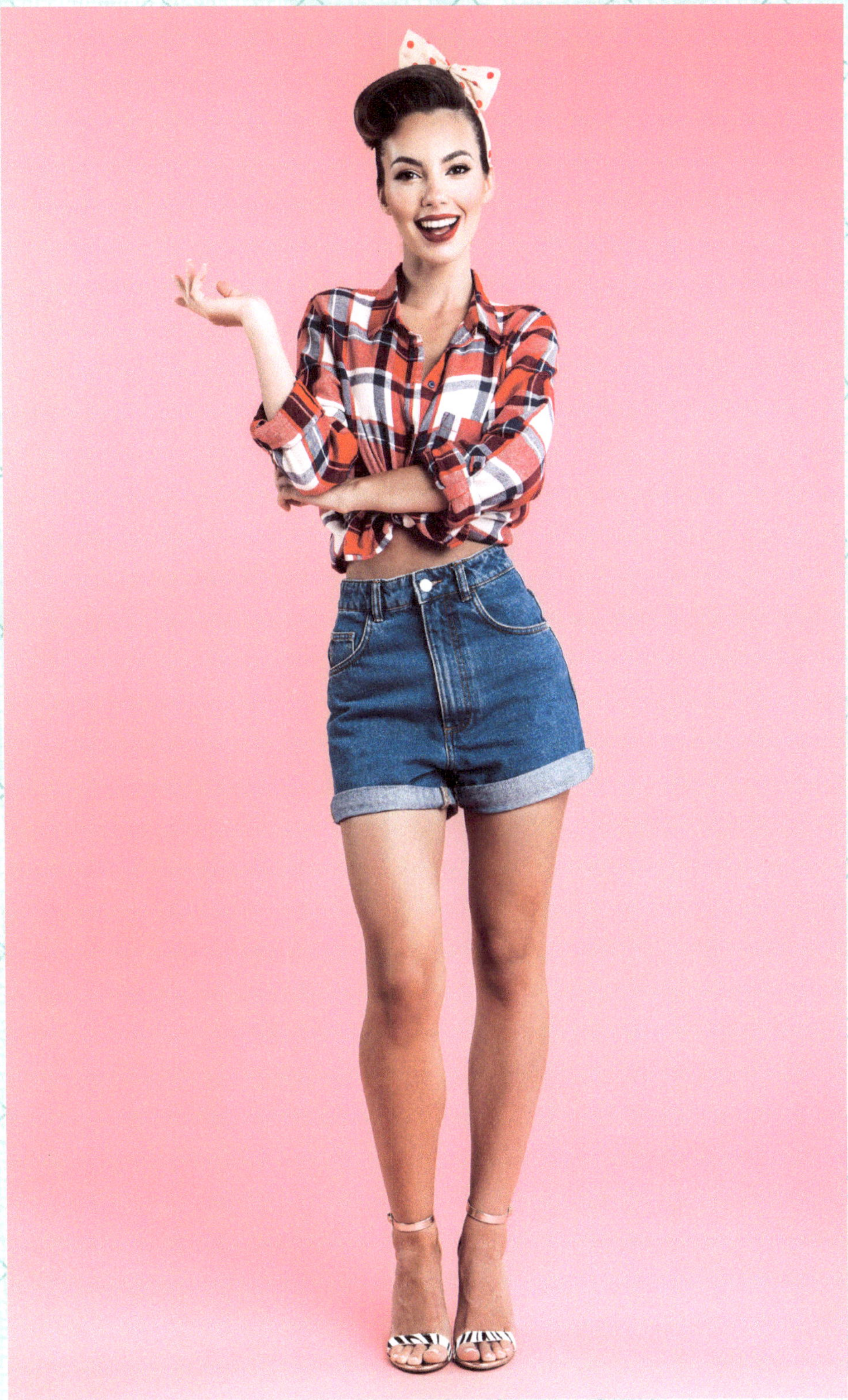

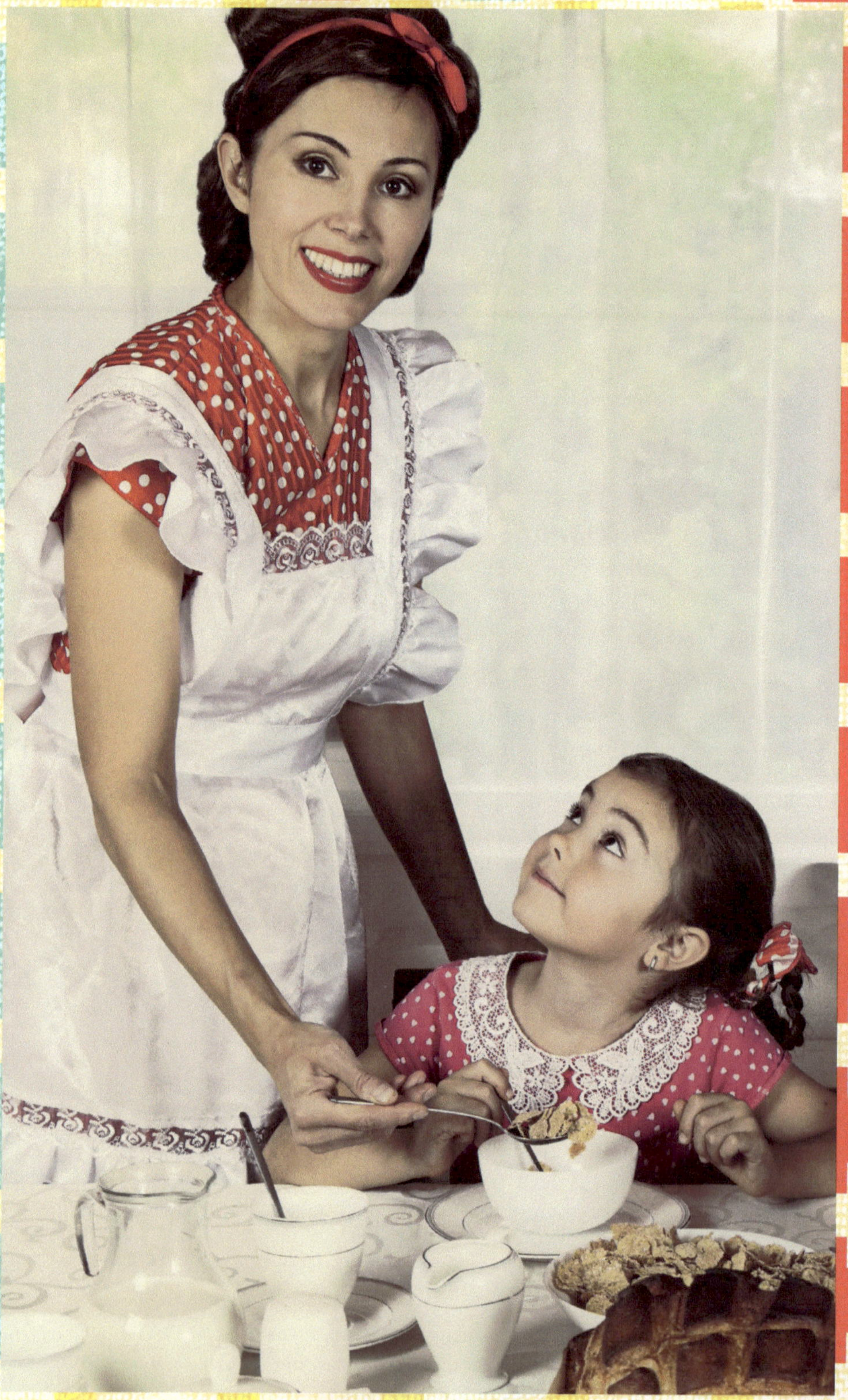

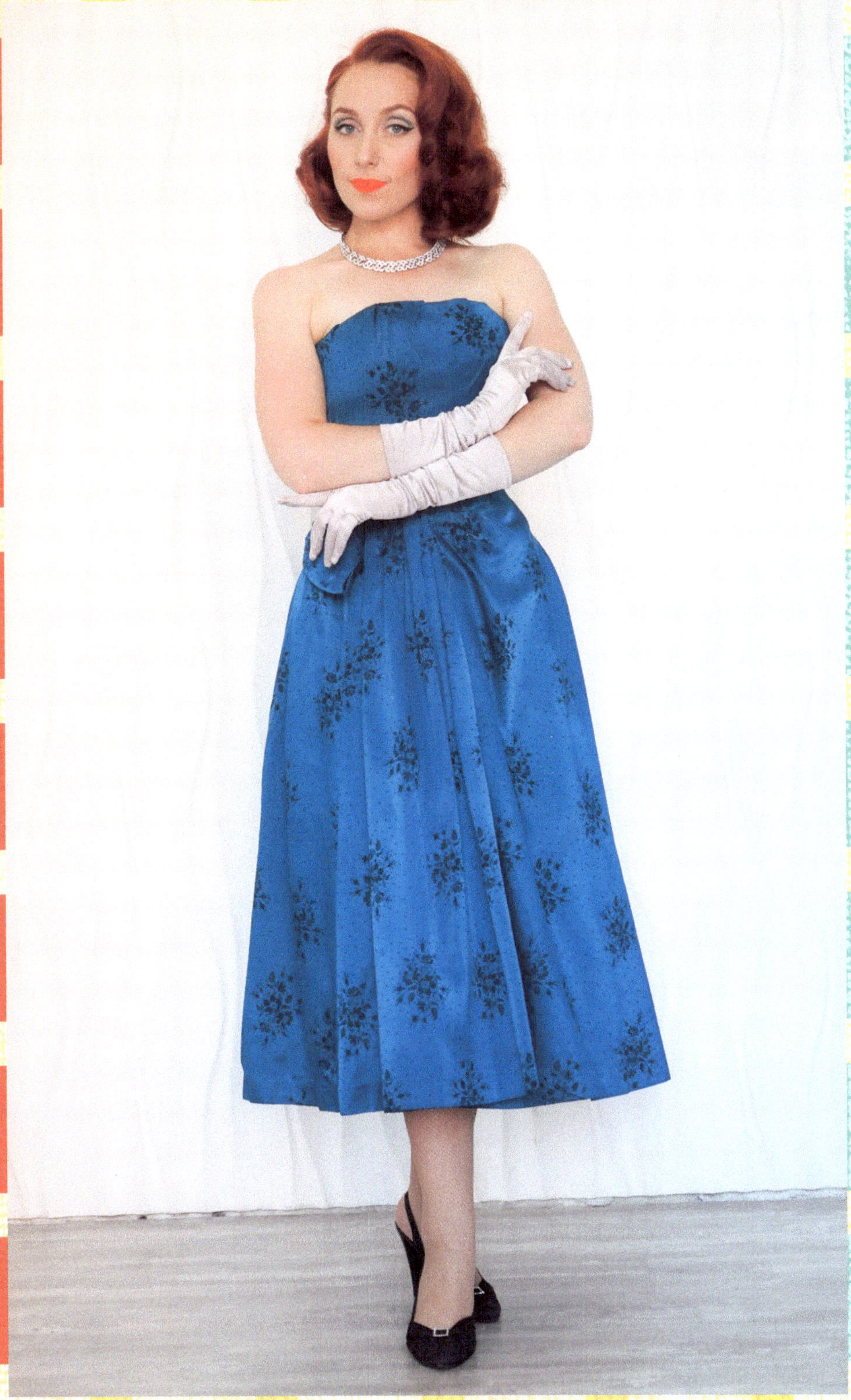

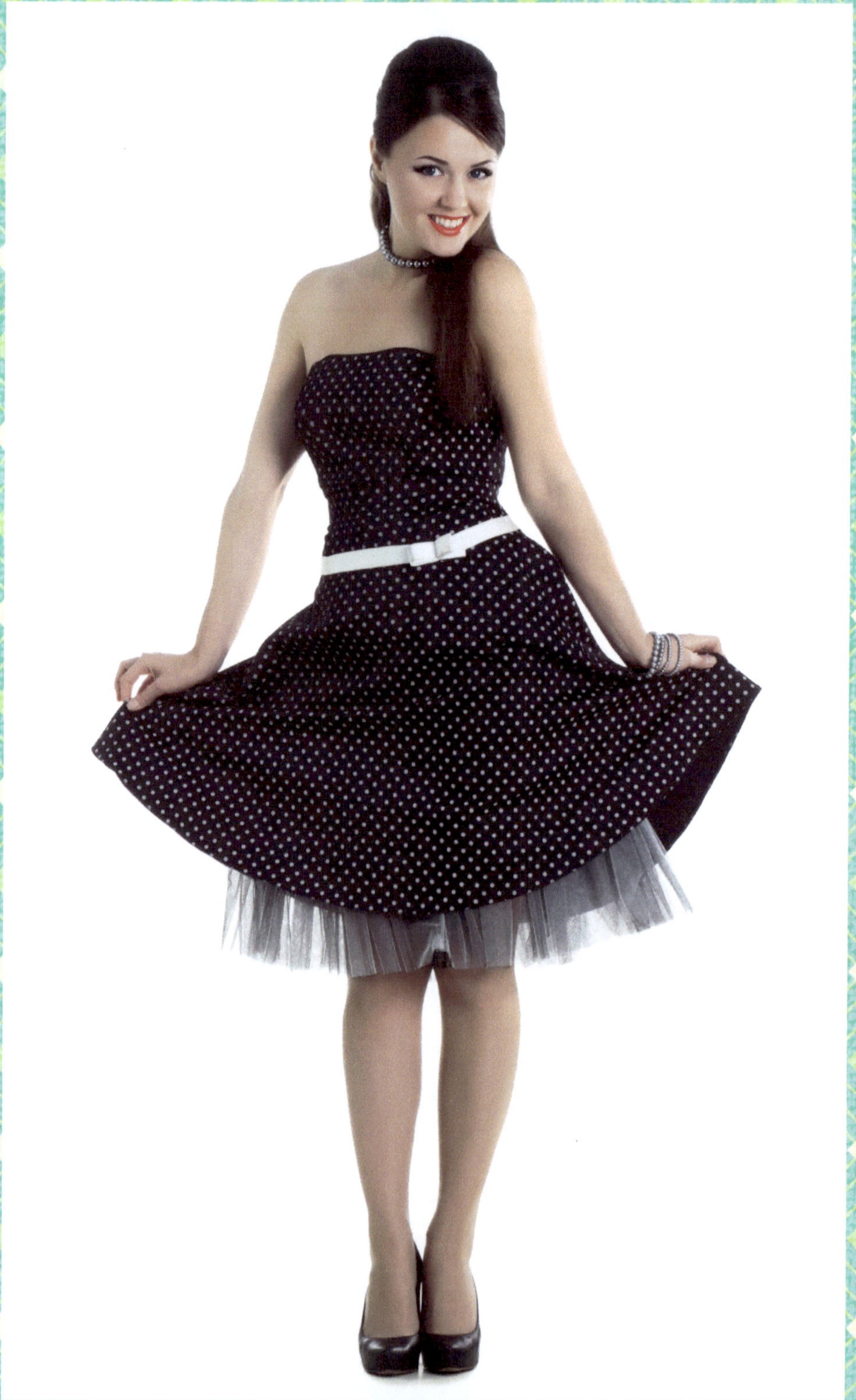

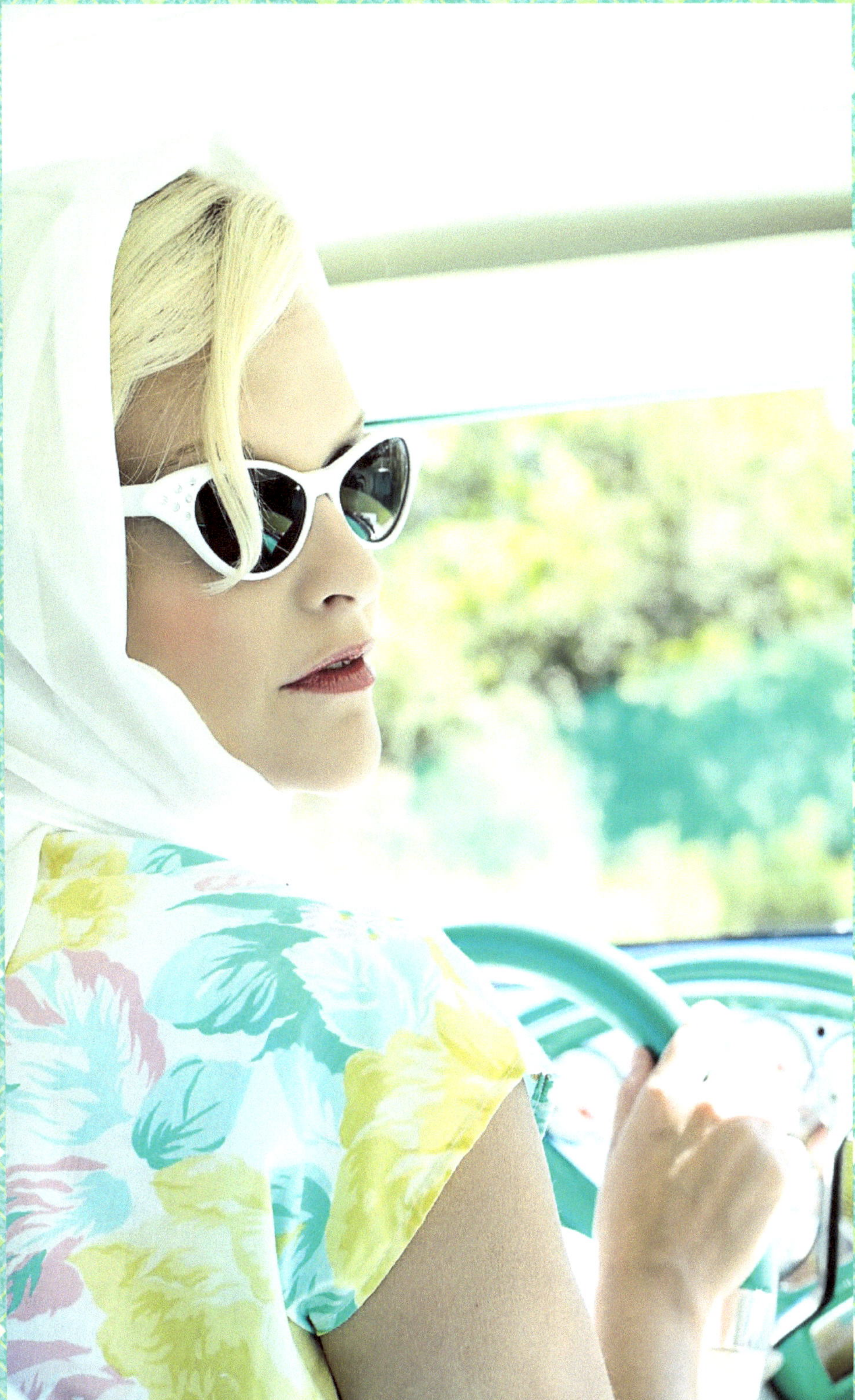

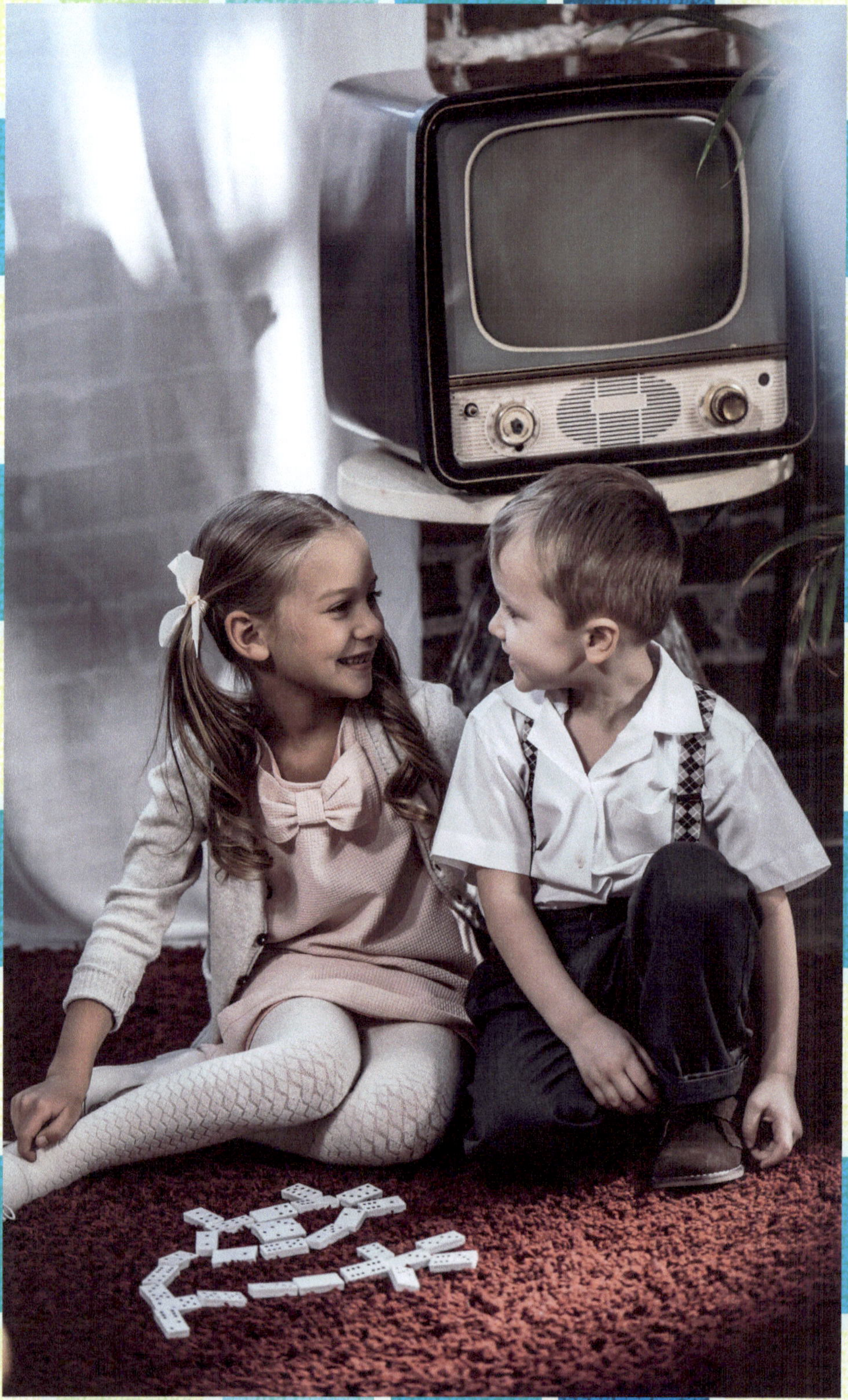

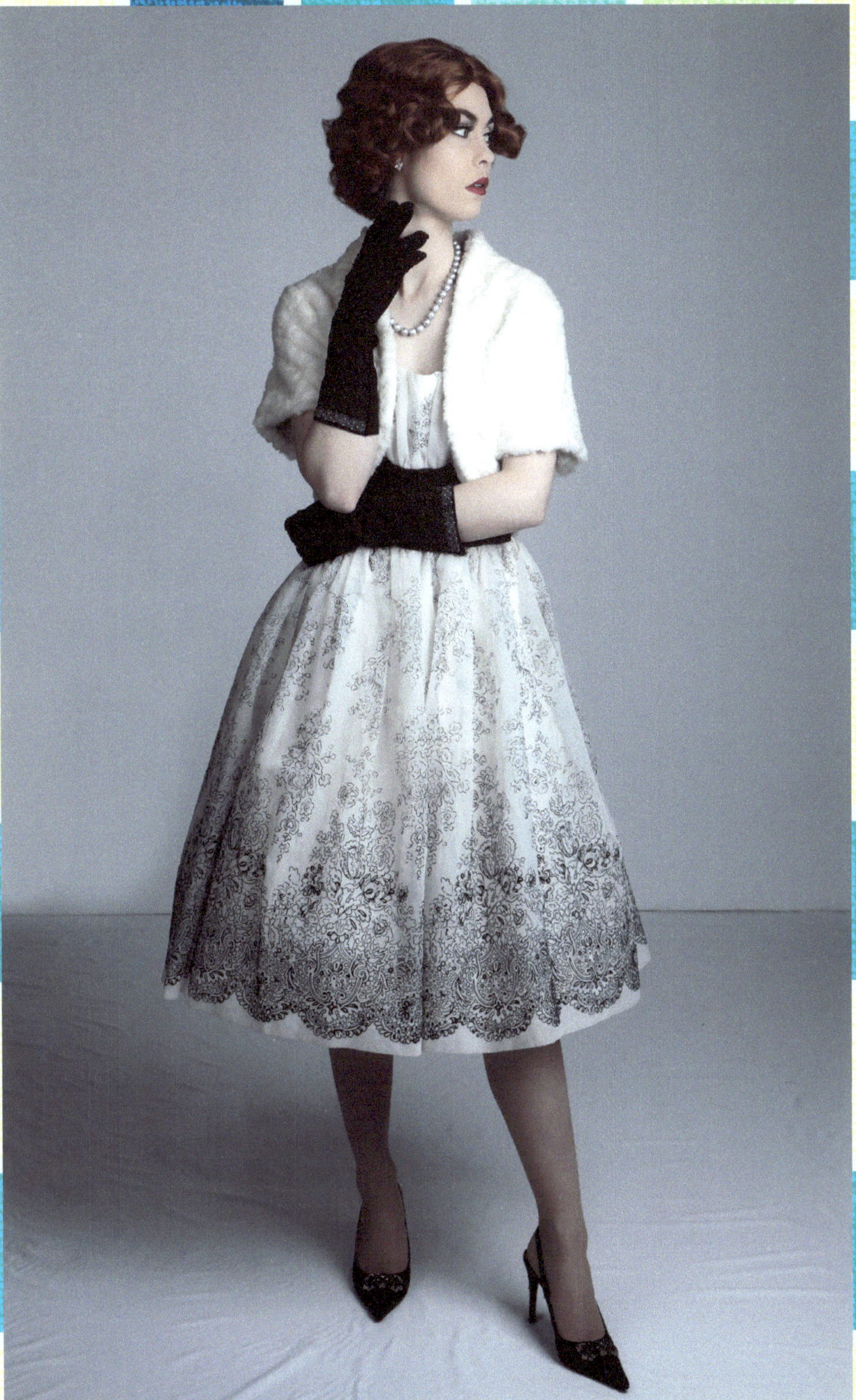

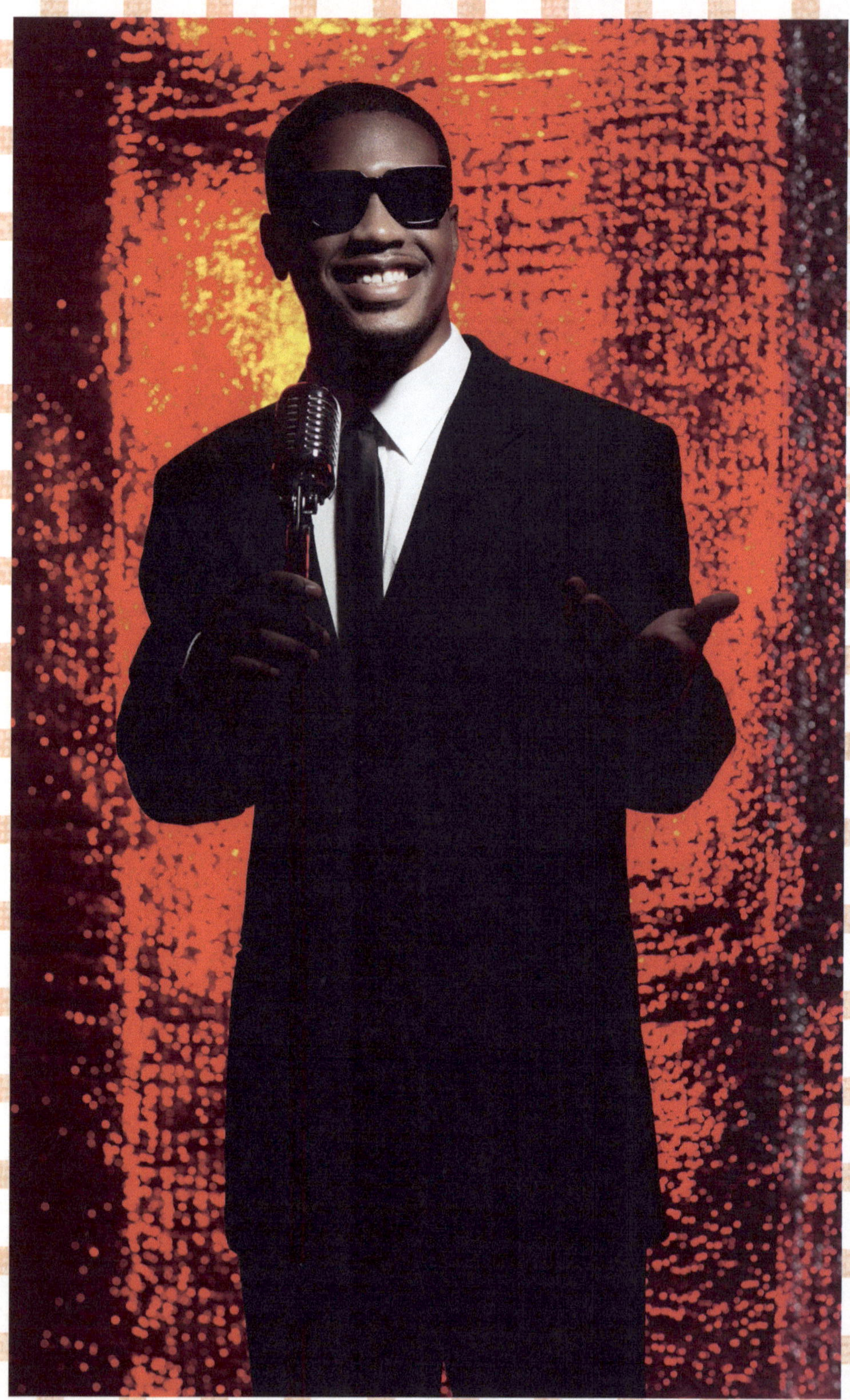

www.ingramcontent.com/pod-product-compliance
Lightning Source LLC
Chambersburg PA
CBHW050847290526
45792CB00002B/554
9798882907333